Cardiovascular Diabetology:
Clinical, Metabolic and Inflammatory Facets

Advances in Cardiology

Vol. 45

Series Editor

Jeffrey S. Borer, New York, N.Y

Cardiovascular Diabetology: Clinical, Metabolic and Inflammatory Facets

Volume Editors

Enrique Z. Fisman   Holon
Alexander Tenenbaum   Tel-Hashomer

23 figures and 5 tables, 2008

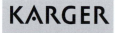

Basel · Freiburg · Paris · London · New York ·
Bangalore · Bangkok · Singapore · Tokyo · Sydney

Prof. Enrique Z. Fisman
Cardiovascular Diabetology
Research Foundation
Holon 58484 (Israel)

Prof. Alexander Tenenbaum
Cardiac Rehabilitation Institute
Chaim Sheba Medical Center
Tel-Hashomer 52621 (Israel)

Library of Congress Cataloging-in-Publication Data

Cardiovascular diabetology : clinical, metabolic, and inflammatory facets /
volume editors, Enrique Z. Fisman, Alexander Tenenbaum.
     p. ; cm. – (Advances in cardiology, ISSN 0065-2326 ; v. 45)
  Includes bibliographical references and index.
  ISBN 978-3-8055-8427-2 (hard cover : alk. paper)
  1.   Diabetes–Complications.   2.   Cardiovascular
system–Diseases–Complications. I. Fisman, Enrique Z. II. Tenenbaum,
Alexander. III. Series.
  [DNLM: 1. Cardiovascular Diseases–complications. 2. Diabetes
Complications. W1 AD53C v.45 2008 / WK 835 C267 2008]
  RC660.C32 2008
  616.4′62–dc22

                                 2007045424

Bibliographic Indices. This publication is listed in bibliographic services, including Current Contents® and Index Medicus.

© Copyright 2008 by S. Karger AG, P.O. Box, CH–4009 Basel (Switzerland)
www.karger.com
Printed in Switzerland on acid-free and non-aging paper (ISO 9706) by Reinhardt Druck, Basel
ISSN 0065–2326
ISBN 978–3–8055–8427–2

To my wife Elsa Meryn Fisman, our daughters Gabriela and Dana, our grand-children Rotem, Guy, Ethan and Einav. To my parents of blessed memory. In gratitude to my beloved family, who in countless ways provides unlimited support, encourages my labor and enriches my existence.

E.Z. Fisman

To my wife, Helena, my best friend and colleague, to our kids, Ilan and Oren who stood by me so strong when I needed them the most. To my mother and father of blessed memory. To a loving family that exceeds my hopes and dreams.

A. Tenenbaum

Contents

Contributors

Professor of Cardiology, Sackler Faculty of Medicine, Tel-Aviv University, Israel. General Secretary, Working Group on Cardiac Rehabilitation, Israel Heart Society; Medical Director, Shfela Region, Leumit Health Fund; Physician-in-charge, field of Cardiac Rehabilitation and Assistant to the Director General, Sheba Medical Center, Tel-Hashomer, Israel.

Director, Cardiac Care Unit, Division of Cardiology, Rambam Medical Center, Bat Galim, Haifa, Israel.

Medical Director, Israel Society for Prevention of Heart Attack (ISPHA), Neufeld Cardiac Research Institute, Sheba Medical Center, Tel-Hashomer, Israel; Professor of Cardiology, Sackler Faculty of Medicine, Tel-Aviv University, Israel.

Department of Nephrology, Wolfson Medical Center, Holon, Israel; Brunner Institute for Cardiovascular Research, Sackler Faculty of Medicine, Tel-Aviv University, Israel.

Professor of Medicine and Cardiology, Universities of Buenos Aires & del Salvador, Buenos Aires, Argentina; Cardiology Consultant, Hospital Militar Central, Buenos Aires; Past-President, Argentine Society of Cardiology, Argentine Foundation of Cardiology, Interamerican Heart Foundation; InterAmerica Representative, Executive Board, World Heart Federation.

Director of Noninvasive Cardiology Unit, Heart Institute, Sheba Medical Center, Tel- Hashomer, Israel; Professor of Cardiology, Sackler Faculty of Medicine, Tel-Aviv University, Israel.

Enrique Z. Fisman, MD .... p. 44, 127, 154

Professor of Cardiology, Sackler Faculty of Medicine, Tel-Aviv University, Israel; Honorary Professor of Cardiology, University del Salvador, Buenos Aires, Argentina; Editor-In-Chief, Cardiovascular Diabetology, BioMed Central, London, United Kingdom.

Ehud Grossman, MD. . . . . p. 82

Professor of Medicine, Vice Dean for Academic Promotions, Sackler Faculty of Medicine, Tel-Aviv University, Israel; Head of Internal Medicine D and Hypertension Unit, Sheba Medical Center, Tel-Hashomer, Israel.

Rogelio A. Machado, MD. . . . . p. 17

Professor of Cardiology and Biostatistics, University del Salvador, Buenos Aires, Argentina; Staff member, Cardiology Service, Hospital Militar Central, Buenos Aires; Chief, Echocardiography Laboratory, Hospital Fancés, Buenos Aires; Member of the Argentine Society of Cardiology.

Franz H. Messerli,
MD, FACC, FACP . . . . p. 82

Professor of Medicine, Director, Hypertension Program, Division of Cardiology, St.Luke's-Roosevelt Hospital, Columbia University, New York, N.Y., USA

Michael Motro, MD, FACC .... p. 127, 154

Full Professor of Cardiology, Sackler Faculty of Medicine, Tel-Aviv University, Israel.

Antonio Paragano, MD. . . . . p. 17

Staff member, Cardiology Service, Hospital Militar Central, Buenos Aires, Argentina; Professor of Cardiology, University del Salvador, Buenos Aires, Argentina.

Roseline Schwartz, MS. . . . . p. 114

Israel Society for Prevention of Heart Attack (ISPHA), Neufeld Cardiac Research Institute, Sheba Medical Center, Tel-Hashomer, Israel.

Marina Shargorodsky, MD. . . . . p. 65

Department of Endocrinology and Diabetes, Wolfson Medical Center, Holon, Israel; Brunner Institute for Cardiovascular Research, Sackler Faculty of Medicine, Tel-Aviv University, Israel.

David Tanne, MD . . . . p. 107

Director, Stroke Center, Department of Neurology and Sagol Neuroscience Center, Sheba Medical Center, Tel-Hashomer, Israel; Professor of Neurology, Sackler Faculty of Medicine, Tel-Aviv University, Israel.

Alexander Tenenbaum,
MD, PhD . . . . p. 44, 127, 154

Director of Research, Cardiac Rehabilitation Institute, Sheba Medical Center, Tel-Hashomer, Israel. Professor of Cardiology, Sackler Faculty of Medicine, Tel-Aviv University, Israel; Editor-In-Chief, Cardiovascular Diabetology, BioMed Central, London, United Kingdom.

Jorge O. Vilariño,
MD, FACC, FAHA. p. 17

Chief, Cardiology Service, Hospital R. Gutiérrez, Venado Tuerto, Argentina; Professor of Cardiology, University del Salvador, Buenos Aires, Argentina.

Reuven Zimlichman, MD. . . . . p. 65

Chief of Medicine, Wolfson Medical Center, Holon, Israel; Brunner Institute for Cardiovascular Research, Sackler Faculty of Medicine, Tel-Aviv University, Israel; Professor of Medicine, Sackler Faculty of Medicine, Tel-Aviv University, Israel.

Preface

The prevalence of obesity, metabolic syndrome and diabetes, which we previously defined as the 'atherothrombotic chain', has reached pandemic proportions worldwide. Consequences of diseases related to this atherothrombotic chain such as hypertension, coronary heart disease, peripheral artery disease and stroke account for much of the morbidity in these patients. As a result, our civilization is currently at war against the threatening enemy of cardio-diabetes. The growing understanding of the inter-relationship between diabetes and cardiovascular disease has been reflected by recent guidelines for diabetes and cardiovascular disease to enhance the diagnosis and management of cardio-diabetes. Indeed, effective cardiovascular prevention in patients with obesity, metabolic syndrome and diabetes needs a global strategy, based on knowledge of the importance of different risk factors, both conventional and newly described. In fact, we are currently witnesses and participants of the emergence of a new scientific discipline – *Cardiovascular diabetology*.

Several independent physiological processes underlie the clustering that defines cardio-diabetes, including insulin resistance, central obesity, dyslipidemia, impaired glucose tolerance, and hypertension. Diabetic arteriopathy, which encompasses endothelial dysfunction, inflammation, hypercoagulability, changes in blood flow, and platelet abnormalities, contributes to the early evolution of these events. Chronic complications of diabetes affecting the cardiovascular system are characterized by a dysfunction of the viscoelastic properties of the arterial vessels and, in particular, of arterial distensibility and compliance. Other nonclassical risk factors such as abnormal oxidized low-density lipoprotein-cholesterol, adiponectin, interleukins, matrixins and C-reactive protein levels are highly correlated with cardio-diabetes.

Although therapeutic improvements and public health policies for risk factor control have brought about a dramatic reduction in cardiovascular mortality among the general population during the last two decades, this success has not been extended to diabetic patients. The presence of diabetes mellitus increases all-cause mortality and, in particular, cardiovascular mortality by 2- to 4-fold. Furthermore, mortality is dramatically increased in the presence of clinical features such as diabetic nephropathy. Although part of this increase can be explained by interaction with other risk factors and by the clustering of diabetes with other risk elements of the metabolic syndrome, increased cardiovascular mortality and morbidity are essentially conferred by the presence of diabetes per se. Atherosclerotic coronary plaques tend to develop earlier and be more advanced and more diffuse in diabetic patients. Unfortunately, the reperfusion strategies have proven less efficacious in those patients. Percutaneous coronary interventions seem to have a worse outcome in these patients, who are affected by a high incidence of re-occlusion. Due to the frequent coexistence of silent ischemia, this diagnosis is often found too late.

Furthermore, a complex of different adverse characteristics of diabetes, including endothelial dysfunction and a prothrombotic state, augments the probability of plaque instability and occlusion. Diabetes renders patients especially prone to heart failure, resulting from both diffuse coronary heart disease and direct microvascular and myocardial damage. Heart failure is the main cause of death during acute myocardial infarction, the global risk of failure being almost three times higher in the presence of diabetes. The risk of developing significant coronary artery disease is also high in diabetic patients because of the increased frequency of dyslipidemia, which is linked to central obesity and insulin resistance.

The complex and intimate relationship between cardiovascular disease and diabetes is discussed in the following chapters of *Cardiovascular Diabetology: Clinical, Metabolic and Inflammatory Facets* in a 'crescendo style' – from basic science to clinical and therapeutic concerns. Beginning with molecular, biochemical, inflammatory and cellular aspects, the book continues with histological and pathophysiologic issues, details particular problems in specific metabolic and clinical settings, and finally analyzes several aspects of clinical pharmacology. The book is made up of nine chapters. In the first, Aronson delineates the biochemical mechanisms by which hyperglycemia induces a large number of alterations in vascular tissue that potentially promote accelerated atherosclerosis. Next, Esper and coworkers clarify how the endothelium is the favorite common target of diabetes and other risk factors, showing that its functional impairment in response to injury occurs long before the development of visible atherosclerosis. Subsequently, Fisman's group describes the main features of interleukins and matrixins, features that suggest a common inflammatory basis for both diabetes and coronary disease. Cernes and coworkers discuss the factors influencing the viscoelastic properties of the arterial wall, Grossman and Messerli analyze the several epidemiological and clinical aspects linking diabetes and hypertension, Tanne analyzes impaired glucose metabolism as a predictor of cerebrovascular disease, and Feinberg's group discuss the impact of metabolic syndrome in patients with acute coronary syndrome. The last two chapters are dedicated to therapeutic issues. Tenenbaum and coworkers talk about the optimal management of combined dyslipidemia, detailing both the classical and modern therapeutic options, and Fisman and coworkers describe the current problems and future prospects of non-insulin antidiabetic therapy in cardiac diabetic patients.

We would like to pay tribute and express our appreciation to the distinguished and internationally renowned co-authors of this book for their outstanding contribution. Despite their many commitments and busy time schedules, these colleagues in Israel, Argentina and the United States enthusiastically stated their acquiescence to cooperate. This book could not have become a reality were it not for their dedicated efforts.

Enrique Z. Fisman
Alexander Tenenbaum

Fisman EZ, Tenenbaum A (eds): Cardiovascular Diabetology: Clinical, Metabolic and Inflammatory
Facets. Adv Cardiol. Basel, Karger, 2008, vol 45, pp 1–16

··························

Hyperglycemia and the Pathobiology of Diabetic Complications

Doron Aronson

Department of Cardiology, Rambam Medical Center, Haifa, Israel

Abstract

Both type I and type II diabetes are powerful and independent risk factors for coronary artery disease (CAD), stroke, and peripheral arterial disease. Atherosclerosis accounts for virtually 80% of all deaths among diabetic patients. Prolonged exposure to hyperglycemia is now recognized as a major factor in the pathogenesis of diabetic complications, including atherosclerosis. Hyperglycemia induces a large number of alterations at the cellular level of vascular tissue that potentially accelerates the atherosclerotic process. Animal and human studies have elucidated several major mechanisms that encompass most of the pathological alterations observed in the diabetic vasculture. These include: (1) Nonenzymatic glycosylation of proteins and lipids which can interfere with their normal function by disrupting molecular conformation, alter enzymatic activity, reduce degradative capacity, and interfere with receptor recognition. In addition, glycosylated proteins interact with a specific receptor present on all cells relevant to the atherosclerotic process, including monocyte-derived macrophages, endothelial cells, and smooth muscle cells. The interaction of glycosylated proteins with their receptor results in the induction of oxidative stress and proinflammatory responses. (2) Protein kinase C (PKC) activation with subsequent alteration in growth factor expression. (3) Shunting of excess intracellular glucose into the hexosamine pathway leads to O-linked glycosylation of various enzymes with perturbations in normal enzyme function. (4) Hyperglycemia increases oxidative stress through several pathways. A major mechanism appears to be the overproduction of the superoxide anion (O_2^-) by the mitochondrial electron transport chain. (5) Hyperglycemia promotes inflammation through the induction of cytokine secretion by several cell types including monocytes and adipocytes.

Importantly, there appears to be a tight pathogenic link between hyperglycemia-induced oxidant stress and other hyperglycemia-dependent mechanisms of vascular damage described above, namely AGEs formation, PKC activation, and increased flux through the hexosamine pathway. For example, hyperglycemia-induced oxidative stress promotes both the formation of advanced glycosylation end products and PKC activation.

Prolonged exposure to hyperglycemia is now recognized as the primary casual factor in the pathogenesis of diabetic complications [1, 2]. Hyperglycemia induces a large number of alterations in vascular tissue that potentially promote accelerated atherosclerosis. Several major mechanisms have emerged that encompass most of the pathological alterations observed in the vasculature of diabetic animals and humans: (1) nonenzymatic glycosylation of proteins and lipids, (2) protein kinase C (PKC) activation, (3) increased flux through the hexosamine pathway, (4) increased oxidative stress, and (5) inflammation.

Advanced Glycosylation End Products

The effects of hyperglycemia are often irreversible and lead to progressive cell dysfunction [3]. For example, in diabetic patients with functioning pancreatic transplants renal pathology continues to progress for at least 5 years after diabetes has been cured [3]. The mechanism for these observations is unclear, but suggests that cellular perturbations may persist despite the return of normoglycemia (the so-called memory effect) [4]. Thus, persistent rather than transient, acute metabolic changes are of pivotal importance in the pathogenesis of diabetic complications.

One of the important mechanisms responsible for the accelerated atherosclerosis in diabetes is the nonenzymatic reaction between glucose and proteins or lipoproteins in arterial walls, collectively known as Maillard, or browning reaction [5] (fig. 1). Glucose forms chemically reversible early glycosylation products with reactive amino groups of proteins (Schiff bases). Formation of the Schiff base from glucose and amine is relatively fast and highly reversible [5] and represents an equilibrium reaction in which the amount of Schiff base formed is dictated by glucose concentration. When glucose is removed or lowered, the unstable Schiff base reverses within minutes.

Over a period of days, the unstable Schiff base subsequently rearranges to form the more stable Amadori-type early glycosylation products. Formation of Amadori product from the Schiff base is slower but much faster than the reverse reaction, and therefore tends to accumulate on proteins. Equilibrium levels of Amadori products are reached in weeks (fig. 1). As with the formation of the Schiff base, the amount of Amadori product formed is related to the glucose concentration [5]. The best-known Amadori product is hemoglobin A_{1C}, which is an adduct of glucose with the N-terminal valine amino group of the β-chain of hemoglobin. Thus, measurement of hemoglobin A_{1C} allows assessment of the degree of glucose control integrated over several weeks.

Proteins bearing Amadori products are referred to as glycated proteins (distinguishing them from enzymatically glycosylated proteins), while the

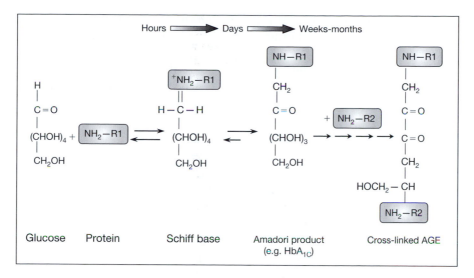

Fig. 1. Formation of advanced glycosylation end-products. The process can be inhibited by aminoguanidine, which reacts with Amadori products and prevents the development of more advanced products. AGE cross-link breakers bind to a fully formed AGE and create a ring prone to a sequence of spontaneous break. The result is a severing of AGE cross bridges between collagen and other macromolecules (see text for details).

process of Amadori product formation is called glycation [5]. Some of the early glycosylation products on long-lived proteins (e.g. vessel wall collagen) continue to undergo complex series of chemical rearrangements in vivo to form complex compounds and cross-links known as advanced glycosylation end products (AGEs) [5, 6] (fig. 1). An important distinction of AGEs compared with the Amadori products is that once formed, AGE-protein adducts are stable and virtually irreversible. The degree of nonenzymatic glycation is determined mainly by the glucose concentration and time of exposure. Therefore, AGEs accumulate continuously on long-lived vessel wall proteins with aging and at an accelerated rate in diabetes [7]. However, another critical factor to the formation of AGEs is the tissue microenvironment redox potential. Thus, situations in which the local redox potential has been shifted to favor oxidant stress, AGEs formation increases substantially [8, 9].

AGEs accumulate in the vessel wall, where they may perturb cell structure and function and accelerate the atherosclerotic process. Glycosylation of proteins and lipoproteins can interfere with their normal function by disrupting molecular conformation, alter enzymatic activity, reduce degradative capacity, and interfere with receptor recognition. AGEs can modify the extracellular matrix, modify the action of hormones, cytokines and free radicals, and alter the function of intracellular proteins [6]. These changes in the normal physiology of the vessel wall are relevant to atherogenesis and may promote atherosclerosis in diabetic individuals.

On of the most important consequences of AGEs formation is their ability to cross-link adjacent proteins. Collagen can become cross-linked because AGEs form covalent heat-stable intermolecular bonds [10]. The amount of cross-linked collagen peptides formed increase as a function of both time and glucose concentration [11]. In contrast to normal cross-links within normal collagen, which occur only at two discrete sites at the N-terminal and C-terminal ends of the molecule, AGEs form cross-links throughout the collagen molecule [7]. Recent studies have demonstrated that collagen cross-linking plays an important role in changing the mechanical properties of tissues, leading to the increased vascular rigidity and the reduced left ventricular compliance in diabetic patients. Collagen cross-linking plays a major role in the pathogenesis of isolated systolic hypertension and diastolic heart failure [12, 13].

Interruption of AGE formation has been shown to ameliorate microvascular and macrovascular complications of diabetes. Aminoguanidine (an analogue of the side chain of arginine), a small nucleophilic compound, is a potent inhibitor of AGEs formation and protein-to-protein cross-linking [10]. The terminal amino group of the compound reacts with glucose-derived reactive α-carbonyl intermediates at the post-Amadori stage (fig. 1). Aminoguanidine has been proven effective in inhibiting AGE formation in vivo in a variety of animal models and clinical studies [5]. However, aminoguanidine is also a NOS inhibitor, which may offset some of its benefits as an AGE inhibitor [6].

Vasan et al. [14] developed a new class of anti-AGE agents that contained a thiazolium structure, which could break α-carbonyl compounds by cleaving the carbon-carbon bond between the carbonyls. The thiazolium agent 3-phenacylthiazolium bromide (PTB) was found to cleave a major proportion of AGE cross-links formed under physiologic conditions. Subsequently, a more stable and more active derivative, 4,5-dimethyl-3-phenacylthiazolium chloride (Alagebrium) was developed for preclinical studies [5]. This agent has been shown to ameliorate arterial stiffness and diastolic dysfunction in both animal and human studies [12, 13].

The AGE Receptor Mediates Oxidative Stress and Inflammation

The pathophysiological significance of AGEs stems not only from their ability to modify the functional properties of proteins, but also to their ability to interact with AGE binding proteins or AGE receptors, through which AGEs elicit several biological phenomena. The cellular interactions of AGEs are mediated through a specific receptor for AGE determinants on cell surfaces [8]. The presence of the AGE receptor (RAGE), a member of the immunoglobulin superfamily of receptors [15], has been demonstrated in all cells relevant to the atherosclerotic process including monocyte-derived macrophages, endothelial cells, and smooth muscle cells [8, 15].

In mature animals, RAGE expression on these cells is low. However, under certain pathological circumstances, sustained upregulation of RAGE occurs. In pathological lesions, abundance of RAGE expressing cells is usually associated with sites of accumulated RAGE ligands. In diabetic vasculature, cells expressing high levels of RAGE are often proximal to areas in which AGEs are abundant [8].

AGE interaction with RAGE on endothelial cells results in the induction of oxidative stress and consequently of the transcription factor NF-κB [16] and increases the expression of adhesion molecules including VCAM–1, ICAM–1, and E-selectin [17]. In addition, engagement of AGEs with their specific receptors results in reduced endothelial barrier function, with increased permeability of endothelial cell monolayers [18]. Thus, the interaction of AGEs with RAGE-bearing endothelial cells can promote initiating events in atherogenesis such as increased lipid entry into the subendothelium and adhesive interactions of monocytes with the endothelial surface with subsequent transendothelial migration.

Binding of soluble AGEs to RAGE-bearing monocytes induces chemotaxis [19], followed by mononuclear infiltration through an intact endothelial monolayer [20]. Monocyte-macrophage interaction with AGEs results also in the production of mediators such as interleukin-1, tumor necrosis factor-α, platelet-derived growth factor, and insulin growth factor-I [20], which have a pivotal role in the pathogenesis of atherosclerosis [21]. Thus, under conditions of enhanced tissue AGE deposition, receptor-mediated interaction of AGE-proteins with vascular wall cells facilitates the migration of inflammatory cells into the lesion with the subsequent release of growth-promoting cytokines.

Schmidt et al. [8, 15] proposed the following two-hit model for RAGE–mediated perturbations in diabetic vasculature. In the setting of hyperglycemia, formation and deposition of AGEs in tissues and vasculature is accelerated. The presence of AGEs (RAGE ligands) in the vasculture results in a basal state of increased RAGE expression and activation (first hit). The superimposition of another stimulus, such as deposition of oxidized lipoproteins or inflammation, results in an exaggerated, chronic inflammation and promotes accelerated atherosclerosis (second hit). In contrast to other inflammatory processes, in which a negative feedback loop terminates cellular activation, RAGE activation appears to result in a smoldering degree of cellular stimulation [8, 15].

The potential role of RAGE in the atherogenic process in diabetes has been demonstrated by Park et al. [22]. In the model of atherosclerosis-prone mice due to homozygous deletion of apolipoprotein E (apoE) gene, the induction of diabetes using streptozotocin resulted in atherosclerosis of increased severity compared to euglycemic apoE controls. The development of vascular disease was more rapid with the formation of more complex lesions (fibrous caps, extensive monocyte infiltration, etc.) and atherosclerosis extending distally in the aorta and major arteries. Increased expression of RAGE and the presence of AGEs in the vessel wall, especially at sites of vascular lesions were also evident. Blockade of AGE-RAGE interaction using a truncated soluble extracellular domain of RAGE resulted in a striking suppression of lesions in diabetic mice, with lesions largely arrested at the fatty streak stage and a large reduction in complex lesions. These effects were independent of glucose and lipid levels [22]. Activation of RAGE-dependent mechanisms contributes not only to lesion formation but also to lesion progression in the same mouse model of atherosclerosis. When established atherosclerosis is already present, RAGE blockade halts the progression of vascular inflammation [23].

RAGE is not the only receptor for AGE–modified proteins that is relevant to atherosclerosis. The macrophage scavenger receptor class A recognizes AGEs and mediates endocytic uptake of AGE baring proteins by macrophages. Although this action does not involve transduction of cellular signals after engagement by AGEs, these receptors may cause clearance and possible detoxification of AGEs [6].

Similarly, CD36, a member of the class B scavenger receptor family, also recognizes and endocytoses AGE proteins [6, 24]. CD36 is not involved in the clearance of AGEs, but induces oxidative stress in the cell [6]. The fact that foam cells in the early phase of atherosclerosis are driven from monocyte/macrophages, in which these scavenger receptors are highly expressed (serving as major oxidized LDL receptors), raises the possibility that scavenger receptors are also involved in AGE-mediated diabetic macrovascular complications.

Protein Kinase C Activation

The metabolic consequences of hyperglycemia can be expressed in cells in which glucose transport is largely independent of insulin. The resulting intracellular hyperglycemia has been implicated in the pathogenesis of diabetic complications through the activation of the protein kinase C (PKC) system [25] (fig. 2).

High ambient glucose concentrations activate PKC by increasing the formation of diacylglycerol (DAG), the major endogenous cellular co-factor for PKC activation, from glycolytic intermediates such as dihydroxy-acetone phosphate and glyceraldehyde-3-phosphate. The elevation of DAG and subsequent activation of PKC in the vasculature can be maintained chronically [25].

PKC is a family of at least 12 isoforms of serine and threonine kinases. Although several PKC isoforms are expressed in vascular tissue, in the rat

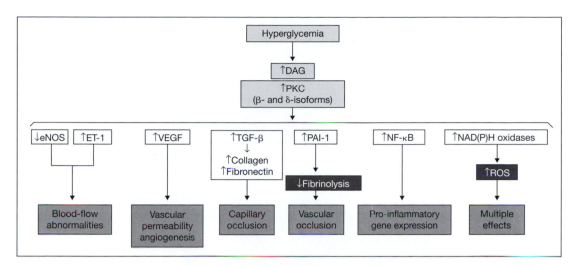

Fig. 2. Consequences of hyperglycemia-induced activation of protein kinase C. Reproduced from Brownlee [38], with permission.

model of diabetes there is a preferential activation of PKC-β_2 in the aorta, heart, and retina, and PKC-β_1 in the glomeruli [25].

The PKC system is ubiquitously distributed in cells and is involved in the transcription of several growth factors, and in signal transduction in response to growth factors [26] as well as nitric oxide [27] and endothelin production [28]. In vascular smooth muscle cells, PKC activation has been shown to modulate growth rate, DNA synthesis, and growth factor receptor turnover [25]. For example, hyperglycemia-induced PKC activation also results in increased platelet derived growth factor-β receptor expression on smooth muscle cells and other vascular wall cells (e.g. endothelial cells, monocyte-macrophages) [29].

PKC activation increases the expression of transforming growth factor-β (TGF-β), which is one of the most important growth factor regulating extracellular matrix production by activating gene expression of proteoglycans and collagen and decreasing the synthesis of proteolytic enzymes that degrade matrix proteins. Increased expression of TGF-β is thought to lead to thickening of capillary basement membrane – one of the early structural abnormalities observed in almost all tissues in diabetes. PKC β selective inhibitor (LY333531) attenuates glomerular expression of TGF-β and ECM proteins such as fibronectin and type IV collagen [26].

PKC activation also appears to be involved in the increased permeability of endothelial cells in diabetes [30], and contributes to endothelial dysfunction by increasing oxidative stress and decreasing NO bioavailability [4, 31].

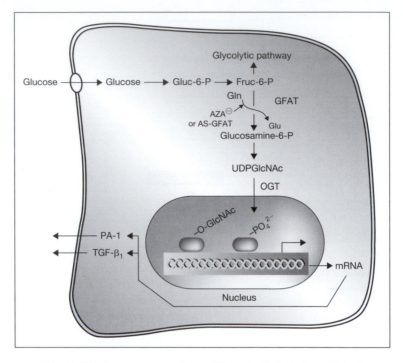

Fig. 3. The hexosamine pathway. The glycolytic intermediate fructose-6-phosphate (Fruc-6-P) is converted to glucosamine-6-phosphate by the enzyme glutamine:fructose-6-phosphate amidotransferase (GFAT). Intracellular glycosylation by the addition of N-acetyl-glucosamine (GlcNAc) to serine and threonine is catalyzed by the enzyme O-GlcNAc transferase (OGT). Increased donation of GlcNAc moieties to serine and threonine residues of transcription factors such as Sp1, often at phosphorylation sites, increases the production of factors as PAI-1 and TGF-1. AZA = Azaserine; AS-GFAT = antisense to GFAT. Reproduced with permission from Brownlee [4].

The Hexosamine Pathway

Shunting of excess intracellular glucose into the hexosamine pathway may contribute to diabetic macrovascular disease. In this pathway, fructose-6-phosphate derived from glycolysis provides substrate to reactions that require UDP-N-acetylglucosamine, such as proteoglycan synthesis and the formation of *O*-linked glycoproteins [4, 32] (fig. 3).

O-glycosylation typically involves the addition of a single sugar, usually N-acetylglucosamine (abbreviated GlcNAc) to the protein's serine and threonine residues. Serine/threonine phosphorylation is a critical step in the regulation of various enzymes, raising the possibility that O-glycosylation might result in perturbations in normal enzyme function.

Many transcription factors and other nuclear and cytoplasmic proteins are dynamically modified by O-linked GlcNAc, and show reciprocal modification by phosphorylation [4, 33] (fig. 3). For example, hyperglycemia increases eNOS-associated O-GlcANc, resulting in a parallel decrease in eNOS serine phosphorylation (which results in enzyme activation) and therefore a decrease in eNOS activity [34]. This pathway is also involved in hyperglycemia-induced increase in the transcription of TGF-β and PAI-1. Inhibition of GFAT, the rate-limiting enzyme in the conversion of glucose to glucosamine (fig. 3), blocks the increase of TGF-β [32] and PAI-1 [35] transcription.

Oxidative Stress

Oxidative stress is widely invoked as a pathogenic mechanism for athero-sclerosis. Oxidative damage to arterial wall proteins occurs even with short-term exposure to hyperglycemia in the diabetic range [36]. Among the sequelae of hyperglycemia, oxidative stress has been suggested as a potential mechanism for accelerated atherosclerosis [9, 37]. Importantly, there appears to be a tight pathogenic link between hyperglycemia-induced oxidant stress and other hyper-glycemia-dependent mechanisms of vascular damage described above, namely AGEs formation, PKC activation, and increased flux through the hexosamine pathway (fig. 4).

Hyperglycemia can increase oxidative stress through several pathways. A major mechanism appears to be the overproduction of the superoxide anion (O_2^-) by the mitochondrial electron transport chain [9]. Physiological generation of O_2 species (particularly the superoxide radical) occurs during normal electron shuttling by cytochromes within the electron transport chain. Hyperglycemia leads to an increased production of electron donors (NADH and $FADH_2$) by the tricarboxylic cycle. This generates a high mitochondrial membrane potential by pumping protons across the mitochondrial inner membrane. As a result, the voltage gradient across the mitochondrial membrane increases until a critical threshold is reached, and electron transport inside complex III is blocked. This increases the half-life of free radical intermediates of coenzyme Q (ubiquinone), which reduces O_2 to superoxide, and markedly increases the production of superoxide [4, 9, 35, 38].

An additional mechanism involves the transition metalcatalyzed autoxida-tion of protein-bound Amadori products, which yields superoxide and hydroxyl radicals and highly reactive dicarbonyl compounds [37]. During Amadori reorganization, these highly reactive intermediate carbonyl groups, known as

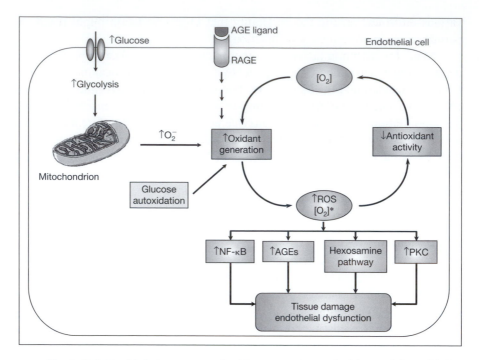

Fig. 4. Relationship between rates of oxidant generation, antioxidant activity, oxidative stress, and oxidative damage in diabetes. $[O_2]^*$ represents various forms of reactive oxygen species (ROS). The overall rate of formation of oxidative products leading to oxidative tissue damage is dependent on ambient levels of both $[O_2]^*$ and substrate. Increased generation of $[O_2]^*$ depends on several sources including glucose autoxidation, increased mitochondrial superoxide production, and as a result of the receptor for advanced glycosylation end products activation. $[O_2]^*$ deactivation is reduced because antioxidant defenses are compromised in diabetes. Note that oxidative stress also promotes other hyperglycemia-induced mechanisms of tissue damage. Oxidative stress activates protein kinase C (PKC) and accelerates the formation of advanced glycosylation end products (AGEs).

α-carbonyls, products which include 3-deoxyglucosone and methylglyoxal, accumulate and lead to 'carbonyl stress' [6, 37].

Some of the individual advanced glycosylation products such as $N^ε$-(carboxymethyl)lysine (CML) and pentosidine are formed in reactions of protein with glucose only under oxidative conditions [39]. Thus, some AGEs are produced by combined processes of glycation and oxidation and have been termed glycoxidation products. Each AGE structure has its own formation mechanism and thus its own dependence on oxidative stress. However, since glycoxidation products on proteins are irreversible, it has been suggested that they may be an integrative biomarker for the accumulated oxidative stress the respective tissue has been exposed to [37]. Indeed, there are strong correlations between levels of glycoxidation products in skin collagen and the severity of diabetic retinal, renal, and vascular disease [40].

Another potential mechanism contributing to oxidative stress involves the transition metal-catalyzed autoxidation of free glucose, as described in cell-free systems. Through this mechanism, glucose itself initiates an autoxidative reaction and free radical production yielding superoxide anion (O_2^-) and hydrogen peroxide (H_2O_2) [41]. This reaction is often catalyzed by transition metals, but even with the catalyst, the reaction is very slow.

Finally, as previously discussed, the interaction between AGE epitopes and the cell-surface AGE receptor upregulates oxidative stress response genes [16] and release oxygen radicals [42]. Thus, hyperglycemia simultaneously enhances both AGEs formation and oxidative stress, and the interaction between glycation and oxidation chemistry can augment each of these processes. Furthermore, oxidative stress generated in the setting of hyperglycemia can lead to the activation of DAG-PKC in vascular tissue [9, 43].

Importantly, all mechanisms of hyperglycemia-induced cellular dysfunction appear to be interrelated and augmented by increased oxidative stress [9] (fig. 4). Nishikawa et al. [9] have shown that hyperglycemia-induced overproduction of mitochondrial superoxide promotes the formation of advanced glycosylation end products, PKC activation, and hexosamine pathway activity. Inhibition of superoxide production by overexpression of manganese dismutase (which rapidly converts superoxide to H_2O_2) or of uncoupling protein-1 (which collapses the proton electromechanical gradients) prevents hyperglycemia-induced superoxide overproduction. Concomitantly, increased intracellular AGE formation, PKC activation, and increased hexosamine formation are prevented [4, 9].

Thus, several seemingly unrelated hyperglycemia-dependent mechanisms that contribute to the vascular complications of diabetes might arise from a single hyperglycemias-induced process: the overproduction of the free radical molecule superoxide.

There is also abundant evidence supporting the importance of reactive oxygen species in inducing and maintaining endothelial cell dysfunction in diabetes. Endothelial cell overproduction of superoxide [4, 9, 38], reduces NO bioactivity because superoxide reacts rapidly with NO, producing the oxidative peroxynitrite radical. In addition to NO scavenging, superoxide overproduction may alter the activity and regulation of eNOS through activation of the hexosamine pathway, leading to reduced eNOS activity [34, 44] (fig. 5).

Diabetes-related oxidative stress also induces DNA single-strand breakage leading to the activation of the nuclear enzyme poly(ADP-ribose) polymerase (PARP). The result of this process is rapid depletion of endothelial energy

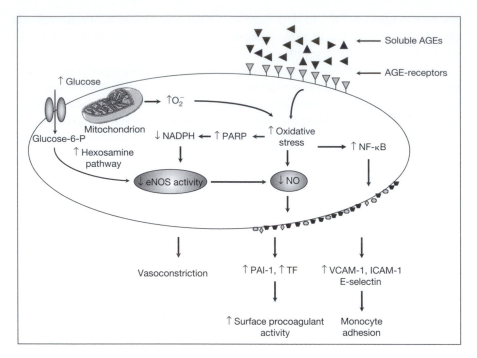

Fig. 5. Mechanisms contributing to increased oxidative stress and endothelial dysfunction in diabetes. Diabetes leads to reduced NO bioavelability and NF-κB activation, resulting in perturbations in vascular tone, increased procoagulant activity and increased expression of adhesion molecules on endothelial cells. TF = Tissue factor; ICAM = intracellular adhesion molecule; PARP = poly(ADP-ribose) polymerase; VCAM = vascular cell adhesion molecule; TF = tissue factor.

sources, including NADPH. Because eNOS is an NADPH-dependent enzyme, it activity is suppressed [45, 46]. A PARP inhibitor can maintain normal vascular responsiveness, despite the persistence of severe hyperglycemia [46].

Diabetes and Inflammation

Chronic, low-level inflammation is an important factor in the initiation and progression of atherosclerosis. Markers of inflammation such as high-sensitivity C-reactive protein (CRP) – a sensitive marker for systemic inflammation – can identify individuals at high risk of developing coronary events.

Increased levels of markers of inflammation such as CRP and interleukin-6 have been documented in both type 1 [47] and type 2 diabetes [48, 49]. Obesity which is commonly present in patients with type 2 diabetes is associated with a proinflammatory state [50]. Another important modulator of inflammation in patients with diabetes is hyperglycemia, which promotes inflammation via AGEs formation (see 'The AGE receptor mediates oxidative stress and inflammation'), but can also induce cytokine secretion by several cell types is hyperglycemia [51]. In monocytes, chronic hyperglycemia causes a dramatic increase in the release of cytokines [52]. Furthermore, recent studies have shown that hyperglycemia, but not hyperinsulinemia, leads to the induction and secretion of acute phase reactants by adipocytes by promoting intracellular oxidative stress [53]. Thus, hyperglycemia might amplify inflammation and promote atherosclerosis and plaque vulnerability.

Insulin-sensitizing interventions such as thiazolidinedions reduced CRP in patients with diabetes [54]. However, the effect of antihyperglycemic therapy on the level of inflammatory markers is more complex. In the DCCT trial of patients with type 1 diabetes, there was a significant reduction of sICAM-1 but no overall treatment effect of intensive insulin regimen on CRP level. Furthermore, there was a significant rise in CRP levels among intensively treated patients who gained the most weight [55]. Thus, given the robust proinflammatory effect of obesity [50], weight gain may mitigate the beneficial effect of intensive insulin therapy on inflammation.

References

1   Laakso M: Hyperglycemia and cardiovascular disease in type 2 diabetes. Diabetes 1999;48: 937–942.
2   Aronson D, Rayfield EJ: How hyperglycemia promotes atherosclerosis: molecular mechanisms. Cardiovasc Diabetol 2002;1:1.
3   Fioretto P, Steffes MW, Sutherland DE, Goetz FC, Mauer M: Reversal of lesions of diabetic nephropathy after pancreas transplantation [see comments]. N Engl J Med 1998;339: 69–75.
4   Brownlee M: Biochemistry and molecular cell biology of diabetic complications. Nature 2001;414: 813–820.
5   Ulrich P, Cerami A: Protein glycation, diabetes, and aging. Recent Prog Horm Res 2001;56:1–21.
6   Goldin A, Beckman JA, Schmidt AM, Creager MA: Advanced glycation end products: sparking the development of diabetic vascular injury. Circulation 2006;114:597–605.
7   Brownlee M, Cerami A, Vlassara H: Advanced glycosylation end products in tissue and the biochemical basis of diabetic complications. N Engl J Med 1988;318:1315–1321.
8   Schmidt AM, Yan SD, Wautier JL, Stern D: Activation of receptor for advanced glycation end products: a mechanism for chronic vascular dysfunction in diabetic vasculopathy and atherosclerosis. Circ Res 1999;84:489–497.
9   Nishikawa T, Edelstein D, Du XL, Yamagishi S, Matsumura T, Kaneda Y, Yorek MA, Beebe D, Oates PJ, Hammes HP, Giardino I, Brownlee M: Normalizing mitochondrial superoxide production blocks three pathways of hyperglycaemic damage. Nature 2000;404:787–790.
10   Brownlee M, Vlassara H, Kooney A, Ulrich P, Cerami A: Aminoguanidine prevents diabetes-induced arterial wall protein cross-linking. Science 1986;232:1629–1632.
11   Monnier VM, Bautista O, Kenny D, Sell DR, Fogarty J, Dahms W, Cleary PA, Lachin J, Genuth S: Skin collagen glycation, glycoxidation, and crosslinking are lower in subjects with long-term

intensive versus conventional therapy of type 1 diabetes: relevance of glycated collagen products versus HbA1c as markers of diabetic complications. DCCT Skin Collagen Ancillary Study Group. Diabetes Control and Complications Trial. Diabetes 1999;48:870–880.

12   Aronson D: Cross-linking of glycated collagen in the pathogenesis of arterial and myocardial stiffening of aging and diabetes. J Hypertens 2003;21:3–12.

13   Aronson D: Pharmacological prevention of cardiovascular aging: targeting the Maillard reaction. Br J Pharmacol 2004;142:1055–1058.

14   Vasan S, Zhang X, Zhang X, Kapurniotu A, Bernhagen J, Teichberg S, Basgen J, Wagle D, Shih D, Terlecky I, Bucala R, Cerami A, Egan J, Ulrich P: An agent cleaving glucose-derived protein crosslinks in vitro and in vivo [see comments]. Nature 1996;382:275–278.

15   Schmidt AM, Yan SD, Yan SF, Stern DM: The multiligand receptor RAGE as a progression factor amplifying immune and inflammatory responses. J Clin Invest 2001;108:949–955.

16   Yan SD, Schmidt AM, Anderson GM, Zhang J, Brett J, Zou YS, Pinsky D, Stern D: Enhanced cellular oxidant stress by the interaction of advanced glycation end products with their receptors/binding proteins. J Biol Chem 1994;269:9889–9897.

17   Basta G, Lazzerini G, Massaro M, Simoncini T, Tanganelli P, Fu C, Kislinger T, Stern DM, Schmidt AM, De Caterina R: Advanced glycation end products activate endothelium through signal-transduction receptor RAGE: a mechanism for amplification of inflammatory responses. Circulation 2002;105:816–822.

18   Wautier JL, Zoukourian C, Chappey O, Wautier MP, Guillausseau PJ, Cao R, Hori O, Stern D, Schmidt AM: Receptor-mediated endothelial cell dysfunction in diabetic vasculopathy: soluble receptor for advanced glycation end products blocks hyperpermeability in diabetic rats. J Clin Invest 1996;97:238–243.

19   Schmidt AM, Yan SD, Brett J, Mora R, Nowygrod R, Stern D: Regulation of human mononuclear phagocyte migration by cell surface-binding proteins for advanced glycation end products. J Clin Invest 1993;91:2155–2168.

20   Kirstein M, Brett J, Radoff S, Ogawa S, Stern D, Vlassara H: Advanced protein glycosylation induces transendothelial human monocyte chemotaxis and secretion of platelet-derived growth factor: role in vascular disease of diabetes and aging. Proc Natl Acad Sci USA 1990;87: 9010–9014.

21   Ross R: Atherosclerosis: an inflammatory disease [see comments]. N Engl J Med 1999;340: 115–126.

22   Park L, Raman KG, Lee KJ, Lu Y, Ferran LJ Jr, Chow WS, Stern D, Schmidt AM: Suppression of accelerated diabetic atherosclerosis by the soluble receptor for advanced glycation endproducts. Nat Med 1998;4:1025–1031.

23   Bucciarelli LG, Wendt T, Qu W, Lu Y, Lalla E, Rong LL, Goova MT, Moser B, Kislinger T, Lee DC, Kashyap Y, Stern DM, Schmidt AM: RAGE blockade stabilizes established atherosclerosis in diabetic apolipoprotein E-null mice. Circulation 2002;106:2827–2835.

24   Ohgami N, Nagai R, Ikemoto M, Arai H, Kuniyasu A, Horiuchi S, Nakayama H: Cd36, a member of the class b scavenger receptor family, as a receptor for advanced glycation end products. J Biol Chem 2001;276:3195–3202.

25   Koya D, King GL: Protein kinase C activation and the development of diabetic complications. Diabetes 1998;47:859–866.

26   Koya D, Haneda M, Nakagawa H, Isshiki K, Sato H, Maeda S, Sugimoto T, Yasuda H, Kashiwagi A, Ways DK, King GL, Kikkawa R: Amelioration of accelerated diabetic mesangial expansion by treatment with a PKC beta inhibitor in diabetic db/db mice, a rodent model for type 2 diabetes. FASEB J 2000;14:439–447.

27   Kuboki K, Jiang ZY, Takahara N, Ha SW, Igarashi M, Yamauchi T, Feener EP, Herbert TP, Rhodes CJ, King GL: Regulation of endothelial constitutive nitric oxide synthase gene expression in endothelial cells and in vivo: a specific vascular action of insulin. Circulation 2000;101: 676–681.

28   Park JY, Takahara N, Gabriele A, Chou E, Naruse K, Suzuma K, Yamauchi T, Ha SW, Meier M, Rhodes CJ, King GL: Induction of endothelin-1 expression by glucose: an effect of protein kinase C activation. Diabetes 2000;49:1239–1248.

29   Inaba T, Ishibashi S, Gotoda T, Kawamura M, Morino N, Nojima Y, Kawakami M, Yazaki Y, Yamada N: Enhanced expression of platelet-derived growth factor-beta receptor by high glu-

cose: involvement of platelet-derived growth factor in diabetic angiopathy. Diabetes 1996;45: 507–512.

30   Yuan SY, Ustinova EE, Wu MH, Tinsley JH, Xu W, Korompai FL, Taulman AC: Protein kinase C activation contributes to microvascular barrier dysfunction in the heart at early stages of diabetes. Circ Res 2000;87:412–417.

31   Beckman JA, Creager MA, Libby P: Diabetes and atherosclerosis: epidemiology, pathophysiology, and management. JAMA 2002;287:2570–2581.

32   Kolm-Litty V, Sauer U, Nerlich A, Lehmann R, Schleicher ED: High glucose-induced transforming growth factor beta1 production is mediated by the hexosamine pathway in porcine glomerular mesangial cells. J Clin Invest 1998;101:160–169.

33   Wells L, Vosseller K, Hart GW: Glycosylation of nucleocytoplasmic proteins: signal transduction and O-GlcNAc. Science 2001;291:2376–2378.

34   Du XL, Edelstein D, Dimmeler S, Ju Q, Sui C, Brownlee M: Hyperglycemia inhibits endothelial nitric oxide synthase activity by posttranslational modification at the Akt site. J Clin Invest 2001;108:1341–1348.

35   Du XL, Edelstein D, Rossetti L, Fantus IG, Goldberg H, Ziyadeh F, Wu J, Brownlee M: Hyperglycemia-induced mitochondrial superoxide overproduction activates the hexosamine pathway and induces plasminogen activator inhibitor-1 expression by increasing Sp1 glycosylation. Proc Natl Acad Sci USA 2000;97:12222–12226.

36   Pennathur S, Wagner JD, Leeuwenburgh C, Litwak KN, Heinecke JW: A hydroxyl radical-like species oxidizes cynomolgus monkey artery wall proteins in early diabetic vascular disease. J Clin Invest 2001;107:853–860.

37   Baynes JW, Thorpe SR: Role of oxidative stress in diabetic complications: a new perspective on an old paradigm. Diabetes 1999;48:1–9.

38   Brownlee M: The pathobiology of diabetic complications: a unifying mechanism. Diabetes 2005;54:1615–1625.

39   Wells-Knecht MC, Thorpe SR, Baynes JW: Pathways of formation of glycoxidation products during glycation of collagen. Biochemistry 1995;34:15134–15141.

40   Beisswenger PJ, Moore LL, Brinck-Johnsen T, Curphey TJ: Increased collagen-linked pentosidine levels and advanced glycosylation end products in early diabetic nephropathy. J Clin Invest 1993;92:212–217.

41   Wolff SP: Diabetes mellitus and free radicals: free radicals, transition metals and oxidative stress in the aetiology of diabetes mellitus and complications. Br Med Bull 1993;49:642–652.

42   Yan SD, Chen X, Schmidt AM, Brett J, Godman G, Zou YS, Scott CW, Caputo C, Frappier T, Smith MA, et al: Glycated tau protein in Alzheimer disease: a mechanism for induction of oxidant stress. Proc Natl Acad Sci USA 1994;91:7787–7791.

43   Konishi H, Tanaka M, Takemura Y, Matsuzaki H, Ono Y, Kikkawa U, Nishizuka Y: Activation of protein kinase C by tyrosine phosphorylation in response to H_2O_2. Proc Natl Acad Sci USA 1997;94:11233–11237.

44   Guzik TJ, Mussa S, Gastaldi D, Sadowski J, Ratnatunga C, Pillai R, Channon KM: Mechanisms of increased vascular superoxide production in human diabetes mellitus: role of NAD(P)H oxidase and endothelial nitric oxide synthase. Circulation 2002;105:1656–1662.

45   Garcia Soriano F, Virag L, Jagtap P, Szabo E, Mabley JG, Liaudet L, Marton A, Hoyt DG, Murthy KG, Salzman AL, Southan GJ, Szabo C: Diabetic endothelial dysfunction: the role of poly(ADP-ribose) polymerase activation. Nat Med 2001;7:108–113.

46   Soriano FG, Pacher P, Mabley J, Liaudet L, Szabo C: Rapid reversal of the diabetic endothelial dysfunction by pharmacological inhibition of poly(ADP-ribose) polymerase. Circ Res 2001;89: 684–691.

47   Devaraj S, Glaser N, Griffen S, Wang-Polagruto J, Miguelino E, Jialal I: Increased monocytic activity and biomarkers of inflammation in patients with type 1 diabetes. Diabetes 2006;55:774–779.

48   Aronson D, Bartha P, Zinder O, Kerner A, Shitman E, Markiewicz W, Brook GJ, Levy Y: Association between fasting glucose and C-reactive protein in middle-aged subjects. Diabet Med 2004;21:39–44.

49   de Rekeneire N, Peila R, Ding J, Colbert LH, Visser M, Shorr RI, Kritchevsky SB, Kuller LH, Strotmeyer ES, Schwartz AV, Vellas B, Harris TB: Diabetes, hyperglycemia, and inflammation

in older individuals: the health, aging and body composition study. Diabetes Care 2006;29: 1902–1908.

50 Wellen KE, Hotamisligil GS: Inflammation, stress, and diabetes. J Clin Invest 2005;115: 1111–1119.

51 Esposito K, Nappo F, Marfella R, Giugliano G, Giugliano F, Ciotola M, Quagliaro L, Ceriello A, Giugliano D: Inflammatory cytokine concentrations are acutely increased by hyperglycemia in humans: role of oxidative stress. Circulation 2002;106:2067–2072.

52 Guha M, Bai W, Nadler JL, Natarajan R: Molecular mechanisms of tumor necrosis factor alpha gene expression in monocytic cells via hyperglycemia-induced oxidant stress-dependent and -independent pathways. J Biol Chem 2000;275:17728–17739.

53 Lin Y, Berg AH, Iyengar P, Lam TK, Giacca A, Combs TP, Rajala MW, Du X, Rollman B, Li W, Hawkins M, Barzilai N, Rhodes CJ, Fantus IG, Brownlee M, Scherer PE: The hyperglycemia-induced inflammatory response in adipocytes: the role of reactive oxygen species. J Biol Chem 2005;280:4617–4626.

54 Pfutzner A, Marx N, Lubben G, Langenfeld M, Walcher D, Konrad T, Forst T: Improvement of cardiovascular risk markers by pioglitazone is independent from glycemic control: results from the pioneer study. J Am Coll Cardiol 2005;45:1925–1931.

55 Schaumberg DA, Glynn RJ, Jenkins AJ, Lyons TJ, Rifai N, Manson JE, Ridker PM, Nathan DM: Effect of intensive glycemic control on levels of markers of inflammation in type 1 diabetes mellitus in the diabetes control and complications trial. Circulation 2005;111:2446–2453.

Doron Aronson, MD
Department of Cardiology, Rambam Medical Center
POB 9602
Haifa 31096 (Israel)
Tel. +972 48 542 790, Fax +972 48 542 176, E-Mail d_aronson@rambam.health.gov.il

Fisman EZ, Tenenbaum A (eds): Cardiovascular Diabetology: Clinical, Metabolic and Inflammatory
Facets. Adv Cardiol. Basel, Karger, 2008, vol 45, pp 17–43

....

Endothelial Dysfunction in Normal and Abnormal Glucose Metabolism

Ricardo J. Esper   Jorge O. Vilariño   Rogelio A. Machado   Antonio Paragano

University del Salvador, Buenos Aires, Argentina

Abstract

The endothelium is the common target of all cardiovascular risk factors, and functional impairment of the vascular endothelium in response to injury occurs long before the development of visible atherosclerosis.

The endothelial cell behaves as a receptor-effector structure which senses different physical or chemical stimuli that occur inside the vessel and, therefore, modifies the vessel shape or releases the necessary products to counteract the effect of the stimulus and maintain homeostasis. The endothelium is capable of producing a large variety of different molecules which act as agonists and antagonists, therefore balancing their effects in opposite directions. When endothelial cells lose their ability to maintain this delicate balance, the conditions are given for the endothelium to be invaded by lipids and leukocytes (monocytes and T lymphocytes). The inflammatory response is incited and fatty streaks appear, the first step in the formation of the atheromatous plaque. If the situation persists, fatty streaks progress and the resultant plaques are exposed to rupture and set the conditions for thrombogenesis and vascular occlusion.

Oxidant products are produced as a consequence of normal aerobic metabolism. These molecules are highly reactive with other biological molecules and are referred as reactive oxygen species (ROS). Under normal physiological conditions, ROS production is balanced by an efficient system of antioxidants, molecules that are capable of neutralizing them and thereby preventing oxidant damage. In pathological states, ROS may be present in relative excess. This shift of balance in favor of oxidation, termed 'oxidative stress', may have detrimental effects on cellular and tissue function, and cardiovascular risk factors generate oxidative stress.

Both type 1 (insulin-dependent) and type 2 (non-insulin-dependent) diabetic patients have mostly been described under enhanced oxidative stress, and both conditions are known to be powerful and independent risk factors for coronary heart disease, stroke, and peripheral arterial disease. Hyperglycemia causes glycosylation of proteins and phospholipids, thus increasing intracellular oxidative stress. Nonenzymatic reactive products, glucose-derived Schiff base, and Amadori products form chemically reversible early glycosylation products which subsequently rearrange to form more stable products, some of them long-lived proteins (collagen) which continue undergoing complex series of chemical rearrangements to form advanced glycosylation end products (AGEs). Once formed, AGEs are stable and virtually irreversible. AGEs generate ROS with consequent increased vessel oxidative damage and atherogenesis.

The impressive correlation between coronary artery disease and alterations in glucose metabolism has raised the hypothesis that atherosclerosis and diabetes may share common antecedents. Large-vessel atherosclerosis can precede the development of diabetes, suggesting that rather than atherosclerosis being a complication of diabetes, both conditions may share genetic and environmental antecedents, a 'common soil'.

Ever since the endothelium was discovered by microscopic examination, it has been considered to be a lining that acted as a barrier stopping intravascular coagulation. Nevertheless, in the last decades, the recognition of its multiple functions has shown it to be a true regulator of blood flow and tissue homeostasis [1]. The endothelium is the favorite common target of all risk factors, and functional impairment of the vascular endothelium in response to injury occurs long before the development of visible atherosclerosis.

Diabetes mellitus (DM) increases coronary heart disease (CHD) mortality in men and more so in women, abolishing the sex difference between them. Established CHD risk factors do not account fully for the increased CHD or for the loss of sex differences in risk, and interest has been focused on the potential role of endothelium in DM.

Anatomic and Functional Properties of the Endothelial Cell

Basically, the endothelial cell has the same characteristics as all the cells of the human body; cytoplasm and organelles surrounding a nucleus and contained by the cellular membrane. The cell membrane is made of a double layer of phospholipids separated by water compartments and crossed by complex proteins that work as receptors or ion channels. Various contractile proteins cross the cytoplasm: actin, myosin, tropomyosin, α-actin and others, that allow motor activities [2]. Some are organized as structures like the cortical web, the junction-associated actin filament system related to the intercellular unions, and the striated myofibril-like filament bundles or stress fibers (fig. 1).

The cortical web surrounds the internal surface of the sarcolema and is responsible for the cell's shape and elasticity. It is sensitive to changes of intravascular tension and increases its stiffness with increases of intravascular pressure. It also anchors different membrane proteins, among them annexin, which regulates endo- and exocytosis, the E-selectins and cadherin, related to the adhesiveness of leukocytes and platelets. The adherence of these elements and their passage through the endothelial cell depends on the integrity of the cortical membrane.

The *junction-associated actin filament system*, known as the FAU system, is found in the intercellular space and its contraction and relaxation controls the

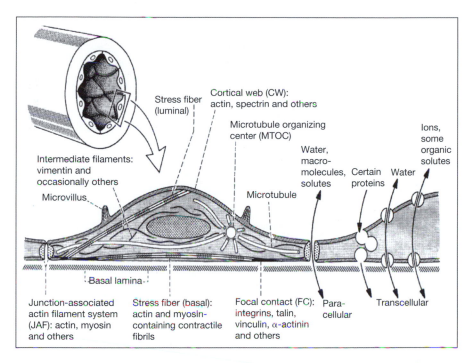

Fig. 1. General organization of the cytoskeleton in vascular endothelial cells. From Drenckham and Ness [2].

dimension of the intercellular space. In this way, it regulates the passage of solutes and macromolecules between the blood and the subendothelial space. It is activated by Ca^{2+} concentrations, intracellular second messengers and the common factor of the external function of cells with intermittent or cyclic activities, the energy being provided by adenosine triphosphate (ATP). Pro-inflammatory cytokines, reactive oxygen species, thrombin, platelet-activating factor, an increase of Ca^{2+} concentration in ischemic conditions, ATP exhaustion and toxic substances, alter the functions of the junction-associated actin filament system allowing opening of the intercellular space and altering the endothelial permeability. The FAU system is closely related to the intercellular adhesion molecules, especially with VE-cadherin, maintaining a balance between adhesive and contractile forces. Both cyclic adenosine monophosphate (cAMP), originated through the adenylate-cyclase, and the cyclic guanine mono-phosphate (cGMP), generated by a Ca^{2+}-nitric oxide guanylate-cyclase dependent pathway, are second messengers that stabilize the FAU system and counteract the induction of intercellular separation, which is done through a Ca^{2+}-dependent calmodulin. Nitrates behave the same way. Protein-kinase C (PKC) activation has the opposite effect (fig. 2).

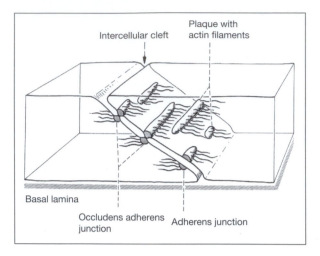

Fig. 2. Intercellular cleft and occludens adherens junction in vascular endothelial cells. From Drenckham and Ness [2].

Stress fibers are myofibril-like straight filament bundles composed of actin filaments interspersed with myosin filaments in a similar way as in striated muscle, and cross the cytoplasm in all directions (fig. 1). The more pressure and friction exerted by the circulating blood, the more abundant are the stress fibers. As with all contracting tissues, their contraction and relaxation depend on the intracellular Ca^{2+} concentration and the presence of ATP; their principal function is to adapt the shape of the cells to the mechanical forces of blood flow and wall distention, reducing the possibility of cellular lesions. When flow increases, so does shear stress and the cells flatten and align in the direction of blood flow, whereas when flow decreases shear stress also does and the cells increase their volume losing their alignment, giving a cobblestone paving appearance.

Morphological changes acquire importance in capillary flow because they can slow or halt flow, as can be seen under the effects of serotonin, histamine, noradrenalin and thrombin, although FAU also acts on this function. In the capillaries, the blood cells are usually larger than the diameter, but flow through the capillary by two main mechanisms: (1) by the flexibility and deforming capacity of both types of cells, blood and endothelial, and (2) by the negative electrostatic charge both cells have and, therefore, repel each other. Endothelial cells have a negative electrostatic charge because of the high concentration of sialic acid. If this concentration is diminished for any reason, blood flow is disturbed.

The cell membrane is covered with flask-shaped membrane invaginations, sometimes shaped like a pocket and sometimes protruding out of the membrane, other times flattened, undistinguished from the basic structure of the cell membrane, but all of them very rich in lipids, sphingomyelin, complex protein structures and multiple receptors. These sites have been called 'caveolae'. They are so abundant that it is estimated that they occupy between 5 and 10% of the total cell surface, and are presumed to be cellular membrane receptor-effector areas [3]. Under normal circumstances there are various ways of transporting plasmatic molecules through the endothelial barrier: (a) intercellular unions that generally act as filters controlled by the hydrostatic pressure that allow the passage of water and dissolved substances; (b) vesicles formed from the 'caveolae' that ease the passage of macromolecules through the cell membrane and cytoplasm, and (c) true transcellular channels usually formed from various caveolae that connect opposite sides of the cell membrane. Through them, the endothelial cell regulates the passage of fluid and macromolecules between the vascular and cellular compartments, and when this fails in the venous capillary area, edema is produced, a situation that can be caused by toxic and vasoactive substances.

Endothelial Physiology

The endothelial cell behaves as a receptor-effector structure which senses different physical or chemical stimuli that occur inside the vessel and, therefore, modifies the vessel shape or releases the necessary products to counteract the effect of the stimulus and maintain homeostasis. The endothelium is capable of producing a large variety of different molecules, which act as agonists and antagonists, therefore balancing their effects in opposite directions. Endothelium produces vasodilators and vasoconstrictors, procoagulants and anticoagulants, inflammatory and anti-inflammatory substances, fibrinolytics and antifibrinolytics, oxidizing and antioxidizing molecules and many others (fig. 3) [1–6]. When endothelial cells lose their ability to maintain this delicate balance, the conditions are given for the endothelium to be invaded by lipids and leukocytes (monocytes and T lymphocytes). The inflammatory response is incited and fatty streaks appear, the first step in the formation of the atheromatous plaque. If the situation persists, fatty streaks progress and the resultant plaques are exposed to rupture and set the conditions for thrombogenesis and vascular occlusion.

Nitric Oxide

Nearly all stimuli that produce vasodilatation do it through nitric oxide (NO), a volatile, biologically active gas present in practically all tissues, which

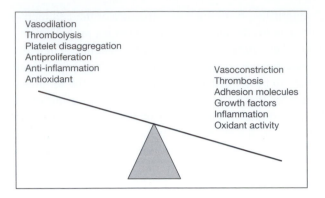

Fig. 3. Regulatory functions of the endothelium. Normal or anti-atherogenic versus dysfunctional or atherogenic properties. From Esper et al. [5].

thanks to its low molecular weight and its lipophilic properties diffuses easily across the cell membranes. The NO crosses the endothelial intima and reaches the smooth muscular tissue of the arterial wall, and, through nitrosylation of the hem from the guanylate cyclase, degrades the GTP-releasing cGMP, which in turn regulates the cytosolic Ca^{2+} and causes smooth muscle fiber relaxation and therefore vasodilatation [7].

NO is produced by the action of nitric oxide synthases (NOS) on the amino acid L-arginine, producing NO and L-citruline, requiring O_2 and nicotinamide adenine dinucleotide phosphate (NADP) coenzyme, essential in redox processes. Tetrahydrobiopterin accelerates this process, which is favored by other cofactors like flavin adenine dinucleotide, and thiol groups like cysteine and reduced glutathione. Three NOS isoenzymes are known, two constitutives and low production, NOS-I from neurological tissue and NOS-III from endothelial cells, both responding to agonists that increase intracellular Ca^{2+}. The other one, inducible NOS-II, is specially expressed in macrophage and endothelial cells due to the effect of pro-inflammatory cytokines and can release several times more NO than the constitutive NOS. Both constitutives and inducible NOS are in the endothelial cells. Constitutive NOS produces NO for short periods when it is induced by vasodilators like acetylcholine or bradykinin. Inducible NOS synthesize NO for longer periods in a constant manner when the stimulus comes from proinflammatory cytokines like tumor necrosis factor-α (TNF-α) [7, 8].

The most important stimulation for NO release comes from shear stress that is caused by the increase in blood velocity and leads to a vasodilatation proportional to the amount of NO released by the endothelium [9]. This vasodilatation is called endothelium-dependent. The endothelial cell membranes contain specialized ion channels, such as Ca^{2+}-activated K^+ channels, which open in response to shear stress [10]. The effect is to hyperpolarize the endothelial cell, increasing the driving force for Ca^{2+} entry and activating the enzyme NOS-III and the subsequent generation of NO [10]. Nitrates given in any way are NO donors, unconfined NO into the circulation directly releasing cGMP in the smooth muscle cell and causing a vasodilatation that is not dependent on the endothelial response, and for this reason it is called endothelium-independent vasodilatation. Shear stress induces a persistent production of NO that maintains a constant vasodilatation [11].

Shear stress explains the importance of the hemodynamic factor in the formation and localization of plaque fissures. These usually develop in areas were the shear stress is low ($<6\,din/cm^2$), oscillating or retrograde, were NO release is diminished and adhesion molecules are increased and chemical and growth factors create a pro-inflammatory atmosphere. On the other hand, a high shear stress ($>70\,din/cm^2$) can cause endothelial erosion and provoke platelet aggregation, or cause plaque rupture or damage. That is to say that a low or retrograde shear stress allows plaque formation and progression of the atherosclerotic lesion, and a high a shear stress causes plaque damage. Physiological levels of shear stress that protect the endothelium are between these two values ($6–70\,din/cm^2$) [12–15].

NO apart from being a vasodilator, also reduces vascular permeability and monocyte and lymphocyte adhesion molecules synthesis. NO also reduces platelet aggregation, tissue oxidation, tissue inflammation, activation of thrombogenic factors, cell growth, proliferation and migration, inhibits proatherogenic and pro-inflammatory cytokines expression and favors fibrinolysis. Nuclear factor kappa-B (NFκB) inhibitor (I-κB) is also expressed by NO. All these factors reduce atherogenesis and its complications. For this reason NO is considered the antiatherogenic molecule [16–22].

The endothelial cell releases angiotensin II (A-II) as an antagonist of NO by means of hydrolyzing angiotensin I by angiotensin-converting enzyme (ACE). Through AT1 receptors, A-II causes vasoconstriction and prothrombogenic, oxidizing and antifibrinolytic effects, also favoring adhesion molecule expression and leukocyte adhesion. It also stimulates growth and proliferation factors, activates inflammation and incites the expression of proinflammatory and proatherogenic cytokines. All of these effects allow atherosclerosis to start its development, progression and complications. A-II also stimulates endothelin converting enzyme that degrades big-endothelin-releasing endothelin I, the most powerful vasoconstrictor on vessel walls [23–25].

As can be seen, depending on the balance of these two substances, NO and A-II, a vasodilator and antiatherosclerotic or vasoconstrictor and atherogenic effect will prevail. This does not necessarily happen by increased production of one or the other, the diminished synthesis of one of them will make normal amounts of the other prevail (fig. 3). The endothelium should maintain an adequate homeostasis so that disease does not appear, and this depends on the capacity it has of producing the protective molecules. When this function is lost or damaged, we refer to it as 'endothelial dysfunction' or 'endothelial activation'. The classical cardiovascular risk factors (hypercholesterolemia, hypertension, smoking, diabetes, sedentary lifestyle, etc.) and the so-called new risk factors like hyperhomocysteinemia, lipoprotein Lp(a), infections by *Chlamydia pneumoniae, Helicobacter pylori, Cytomegalovirus*, herpes zoster virus or *Bacteroides gingivalis*, all have a common property which is to promote a state of oxidative stress that directly or through heating proteins (HSP-60) stimulates NF-κB replication that leads to the production of proatherogenic cytokines like TNF-α, IL-1, IL-6, adhesion molecules, and chemokines that cause inhibition of ONS-III activity and NO production, favoring A-II synthesis and activity [26–30]. The pro-inflammatory cytokines stimulate the replication of NF-kB that leads to more cytokine production. Then, inflammation amplifies the inflammatory response [31].

It is useful to consider the other great source of vasodilatation, via an arachidonic acid cascade that ends in prostacyclins, which release cAMP from ATP that regulates cytosolic Ca^{2+}, therefore producing relaxation and vasodilatation. There are other vasodilator mechanisms, like endothelium-derived hyperpolarizing factor that increases the intracellular concentration of K through CP450 cytochrome, and natriuretic peptide-C intervention. It has recently been postulated that some ACE inhibitors stimulate endothelium derived hyperpolarizing factor which would explain some of the beneficial effects these compounds have that cannot be satisfactorily explained by ACE inhibition only. All these alternative mechanisms are important in certain situations to substitute NO deficit.

Endothelium and Renin-Angiotensin System

The renin-angiotensin system (RAS) is a cascade of enzymatic reactions that ends in A-II. The renin, produced by the kidney, acts on the angiotensinogen produced by the liver degrading it to A-I, which in turn will be acted on by circulating or tissue ACE and hydrolyzed to A-II. Chymase, carboxypeptidase, cathepsin G and tonin can generate A-II from A-I independently of ACE, and A-II can also originate directly from angiotensinogen by nonrenin enzymes, such as tissue plasminogen activator (t-AP), cathepsin G and tonin. Because of its structural similarity, ACE also degrades other peptides that are substrates to this enzyme such as substance P, enkephalins, neurotensin, tachykinin and kininogen, the latter being responsible for bradykinin generation. The stimulation of

ONS-III induces ON synthesis and prostacyclin production, which in turn have opposite effects to those of A-II. As can be seen, the interrelationship between agonists and antagonists is very complex and requires a delicate balance which is the primary function of the endothelium [26–31]. There are two RAS, one is circulatory and the other is in the tissues. The latter, at a cellular level, develops approximately 90% of the activity of the system.

A-II acts by stimulating specific receptors. In the human body we are able to distinguish two different types of receptors: AT1 and AT2. The AT1 receptors are responsible for the known effects of A-II; vasoconstriction, increase in aldosterone activity, myocardial hypertrophy, vessel wall smooth muscle proliferation, renal sodium reabsorption, increase in peripheral noradrenergic activity, vasopressin release, sympathetic stimulation, decrease in renal blood flow, etc. The effects of the AT2 receptor stimulation are not completely known, but there are animal and human data that allow us to assume that they are responsible for apoptosis, a clear inhibition of proliferation, vascular endothelial neogenesis stimulation and vasodilatation, effects that are opposite to those of AT1 receptor stimulation [32]. AT2 receptors are found in the fetus during the last 3 months of pregnancy and during the first 3 weeks of life. In adult tissues, they are predominantly expressed in the brain and adrenals, with lower levels expressed elsewhere [33]. They are expressed when there is vascular injury.

There are different angiotensin peptides capable of stimulating the AT1 receptors with varying intensities: A-II(2–8), A-IV(3–8), A-II(1–7). This fact and the different effects of each one when the specific receptors were blocked suggest that there are other specific receptors sensitive to each of these peptides. In experimental animal models, different specific receptor variants have been isolated and cloned, for example in the rat AT1A, AT1B, and AT1C. Nevertheless, in human beings, only AT1 and AT2 receptors of AT-II have been identified. A-II(1–7) has effects opposite to those of the classic A-II, producing vasodilatation, inhibiting proliferation, myocardial hypertrophy and vascular smooth muscle proliferation, and it is very unlikely that it should act through the known AT1 and AT2 receptors. This led to believe that there are specific receptors for it. This has actually been reported recently although they have not yet been cloned [32–34].

Oxidant Byproducts and Atherosclerosis

Oxidant products, such as superoxide anion (O_2^-), hydrogen peroxide (H_2O_2), hydroxyl radical (HO), hypochlorous acid (HOCl) and lipid radicals [33], are produced as a consequence of normal aerobic metabolism. These molecules are highly reactive with other biological molecules and are referred to as

Table 1. Normal aerobic metabolism oxidizing and antioxidizing systems

Oxidizing systems	Antioxidizing systems
Oxidant byproducts	*Enzymatic antioxidants*
Superoxide anion (O_2^-)	Superoxide dismutase
Hydrogen peroxide (H_2O_2)	Glutathione peroxidase
Hydroxyl radical (HO)	Catalase
Hypochlorous acid (HOCl)	
Lipid radicals	
Enzymatic oxidants	*Lipid-soluble antioxidants*
Dehydrogenase xantine	Vitamin E
NADPH oxidase	β-Carotene
Myeloperoxidase	
Monoamino-oxidase	*Water-soluble antioxidants*
ON synthetase	Vitamin C

reactive oxygen species (ROS). Under normal physiological conditions, ROS production is balanced by an efficient system of antioxidants; molecules that are capable of neutralizing them and thereby of preventing oxidant damage. In the tissues, naturally occurring enzymatic antioxidants such as superoxide dismutase, glutathione peroxidase, and catalase play an important role in the conversion of ROS to oxygen and water. There are several nonenzymatic antioxidants, including the lipid-soluble vitamin E and β-carotene and the water-soluble antioxidant vitamin C, which particularly protects plasma lipids from peroxidation, scavenges superoxide anion, and plays a role in recycling vitamin E [35]. In pathological states, ROS may be present in relative excess. This shift of balance in favor of oxidation, termed 'oxidative stress', may have detrimental effects on cellular and tissue function. As mentioned before, cardiovascular risk factors generate oxidative stress (table 1).

LDL-cholesterol molecules are easily oxidized in a state of oxidative stress, especially the small and dense molecules. Native LDL molecules are innocuous, in the sense that they do not produce inflammatory reactions nor do they lead to foam cell production when phagocytosed by specific native macrophage receptors. Oxidized LDL-cholesterol molecules (LDL-ox), are highly immunogenic, and are associated with the upregulation of pattern-recognition receptors for innate immunity, including scavenger receptors and Toll-like receptors [36, 37]. They are found in all atherosclerotic lesions and generate antibodies that are capable of neutralizing them. LDL-ox attacks the arterial intima and leads to release of phospholipids that can activate endothelial cells [38], induces the production of endothelium adhesion molecules and monocytes attraction [39], has endothelium cytotoxic effects, increases proin-flammatory genes activity and cellular growth factors, provokes endothelial dysfunction, platelet aggregation and metaloproteinase expression, and favors thrombogenesis [40]. LDL-ox molecules are found in the subendothelial layers and help to activate monocytes, which are transformed into macrophages, upregulating their scavenger and Toll-like receptors that then phagocyte them. With progressive accumulation of LDL-ox, macrophages modulate their pheno-type turning themselves into foam cells. Foam cells are the principal compo-nent of the fatty streaks which is the first step in atheromatous plaque formation, and they trigger antigenic reactions in T lymphocytes that initiate or increase the immunological response [41]. Also TNF-α is activated and endothelial cell apoptosis induced, mechanisms that have a close relation with the severity of acute ischemic syndromes [42, 43].

HDL cholesterol and apolipoprotein A-1 have direct antiatherogenic and vascular protective effects. They have antioxidant effects attributed to the binding of transition metals and to the presence of paraoxonase, an enzyme carried predominantly by apolipoproteins A-1 and J, containing HDL particles, which has powerful antioxidant effects. Moreover, they have shown anti-inflam-matory effects, scavenging of toxic phospholipids, stimulation of the reverse cholesterol transport, antithrombotic and profibrinolytic effects and attenuation of endothelial dysfunction [44].

The excess of ROS, especially superoxide anion, can oxidize NO and transform it into peroxynitrite (ONOO), an inactive molecule that can lead to more oxidation. This situation is usually seen when ONS-II activation is induced, and by the high concentration of NO it generates. This also happens with high levels of LDL, especially small and dense molecules that are prone to oxidation. Asymmetric dimethyl amino-arginine (ADMA) exists normally in the body and inhibits NO synthesis by competing with L-arginine. In this way, it reduces NO tissue concentration with all the consequences that this causes, to the extent that many investigators consider it a new atherosclerotic risk factor. Serum levels of ADMA keep a close relationship with LDL-ox concentration and vice versa [45, 46]. ONOO can oxidize tetrahydrobiopterin, a critical cofac-tor for ONS [47].

Long-term treatment without intervals with most organic nitrates is fre-quently associated with a progressive reduction of hemodynamic effects. Nitrates activate vascular NADPH oxidase with incremental O_2^- generation, and these highly reactive molecules oxidize NO to ONOO [48]. Moreover, con-tinuous treatment with nitrates causes ONS-III dysfunction by oxidative stress. Reduced bioavailability of tetrahydrobiopterin is involved in the pathogenesis of this phenomenon and is prevented by supplemental folic acid administration. ROS transform regular ONS-III function, and produce O_2^- in place of NO [49].

Oxidative stress may explain the development of tolerance and the impaired endothelial function during continuous organic nitrates administration.

Inflammation and Thrombosis

There is a clear relationship between inflammation and thrombosis, each influencing the other. Inflammatory cytokines induce procoagulant molecules in endothelial cells such as von Willebrand factor, tissue factor and plasminogen-activating inhibitor factors PAI-1 and PAI-2. Activated inflammatory cells also produce molecules that contribute to thrombogenesis, such as tissue factor and thrombin, which in turn generates an intense mitogenic stimulus and platelet activation [50–52]. IL-6 not only increases plasma concentration of C-reactive protein (CRP) in the liver but also fibrinogen, PAI-1, and serum-A amyloid protein. On the other hand, CRP amplifies immunological response inducing leukocyte adhesion molecules and chemokines production in the endothelial cells, and shows synergetic action with bacterial polysaccharides inducing monocyte grow factors [53]. IL-1 provokes synthesis of PAI-1 in the endothelial cells whereas IL-4 induces plasminogen tissue activator (t-PA) by monocytes. Cell surface-based signaling system CD40L ligand (CD154), binding to its receptor CD40 on the leukocyte, can induce tissue factor expression [50]. Platelets can express CD154, the molecule that regulates tissue factor gene expression in the macrophage and smooth muscle cells [51, 52]. As can be seen, this process involves a complex feed-back in which inflammation favors thrombosis, anti-inflammatory treatment has antithrombotic effects, and vice versa [54, 55].

Immunological System and Atherogenesis

Atherosclerosis is related to activation of the immune system [56]. The developing atherosclerotic plaques are infiltrated not only by macrophages but also by T lymphocytes (CD-4)Th called helper cells, and T lymphocytes CD-8, which suggest a specific immunological response [57]. Nevertheless, investigators have not yet reached agreement on whether the effect is harmful or beneficial for the developing plaque. T lymphocytes (CD4)Th1 produce TNF-α, interferon-γ and IL-6, all of them pro-inflammatory compounds that activate macrophages and are responsible for the late hypersensitivity reactions. On the other hand, T lymphocytes (CD-4)Th2 generate IL-4, IL-5, IL-10 and IL-13, all of them anti-inflammatory molecules that promote antibody responses and inhibit macrophage activity energetically [58]. In the atherosclerotic plaque of experimental animals and in humans, inflammatory cytokines produced by T lymphocytes (CD4)Th1, such as interferon-γ and IL-12, have been found in a pro-inflammatory surrounding similar to that of rheumatoid arthritis [59–62]. In other plaques they have not been detected, in which it is suspected that there may be a reduction in the inflammatory response. This fact leads to the belief that the balance between T lymphocytes (CD-4)Th1 and (CD-4)Th2 may play an important role in the progression or regression of the plaque. In this respect, statins play a role modulating immunological activity [63–65].

Sphingomyelinase is another immunological mediator produced by macrophages and endothelial cells when stimulated by inflammatory cytokines. It is one of the substances responsible for oxidized lipoproteins passing through the endothelium, for foam cell formation and progression, and for complications of the atherosclerotic plaque [66, 67].

From Endothelial Dysfunction to Acute Ischemic Syndrome

Atherosclerosis has been considered a disease of 'four concepts'. In a sub-study of 5,209 patients from the Framingham Study followed for 10 years, it was seen that those patients with peripheral vascular disease had more probabilities of having an acute myocardial infarction (AMI) or a stroke, while those who had had an AMI had more possibilities of having a stroke or peripheral vascular disease. Also those who had suffered a stroke had more chances of having an AMI or peripheral vascular disease. From these observations the first concept that atherosclerosis is a diffuse disease was postulated [54, 68].

The finding of lesions in different stages of development throughout the body, even in the same territory, lead to the second concept that 'atherosclerosis is a heterogeneous and multiform disease' [68].

In advanced stages of arteriosclerosis, stage IV and Va by the AHA classification or Ross type III lesion, two types of lesions can be distinguished: (1) Stable or fibrous plaque, with a small and generally central lipid core protected by a thick and resistant cover with a high content of collagen and without signs of inflammation. These lesions usually obstruct the vessel significantly and are easily seen by arteriography. (2) High-risk, unstable or vulnerable plaque, with a large lipid core, usually eccentric, covered by a weak and thin fibrous cap with little collagen and large quantities of macrophage and T lymphocytes that are expression of a great inflammatory reaction that seldom occlude the vessel significantly and is frequently not appreciated by angiography. This has generated the third concept that the 'quality of the plaque is more important than the size', as proved by the fact that these plaques rupture easily and are responsible for the majority of the acute coronary syndromes. According to a meta-analysis by

Falk et al. [69], these high-risk plaques which obstruct less than 70% and even less than 50% of the lumen, are usually asymptomatic, not easily recognized and not considered significant at angiography, though they are responsible for 86% of acute coronary syndromes [68–71].

Classical risk factors play an important part in atherosclerotic disease: high serum cholesterol levels, arterial hypertension, smoking, obesity, sedentary lifestyle and the so-called new risk factors such as hyperhomocysteinemia, Lp(a) lipoprotein, cytomegalovirus, *C. pneumoniae, H. pylori, B. gingivalis*, genetic factors (gene ECA, gene HLA and others), serum inflammatory markers (CRP, serum-A amyloid protein, and others), prothrombotic factors (PAI-I, D-dimer, fibrinogen, von Willebrand, etc.) and microalbuminemia contribute, in different degrees, to make acute coronary syndromes occur. This suggests the fourth concept that 'atherosclerosis is an inflammatory, immunological, polygenic and multifactorial disease' [71–76].

The evolution of the disease can be slow and patients with risk factors may develop chronic or unstable angina or AMI, this form being observed in less than 40% of the cases, or the illness can develop abruptly in patients who were at low risk and asymptomatic when they developed unstable angina, AMI or sudden death. This is found in more than 60% of patients and this fact obliges us to find other explanations based on a new physiopathological model.

All the experience obtained in the last years suggests that the endothelium's dysfunction is not only the initial stage of the atherosclerotic disease that generates plaque formation, but can also cause plaque growth and not protect from high-risk plaque leading to development of a vascular event. Between these two extremes endothelial dysfunction is responsible for all the plaque growth, differences in plaque development and plaque characteristics. For all these reasons, endothelial dysfunction is one of the principal mechanisms in atherosclerotic disease [77]. The presence of classical and new risk factors generates a chronic exogenous state of injury to the endothelium that promotes its abnormal response, vasoconstriction, accumulation of inflammatory cells, migration of smooth muscle cells, increased cytokine production, etc., all factors that help atheromatous plaque formation and in turn generate a negative feedback that leads to a second injury, this time endogenous, that finally leaves the plaque unprotected allowing it to rupture or erode and triggering thrombogenic phenomena [78].

Assessment of Endothelial Function: Invasive and Noninvasive Techniques

Endothelial dysfunction, or loss or reduction of its capacity of defense against proatherogenic factors, is assessed by evaluating any of the endothelial functions, e.g. quantifying circulating adhesion molecules, proatherogenic substances, antifibrinolytics, evaluation of serum markers of inflammation. All these are direct or indirect markers of the endothelium capacity to protect against new atherosclerotic lesions or to protect existing lesions from vascular events. Because of the ease with which it can be done and its reliability, the most commonly used test in basic science and clinical research is the assessment of endothelium-dependent vasodilatation modulated by flow, considered at this moment the gold standard [77].

The first experiments to evaluate endothelium-dependent vasodilatation were performed by invasive techniques catheterizing coronary arteries, where drugs that induce NO release, such as acetylcholine, metacholine, papaverin, substance P, etc., were injected, and the percentage of vasodilatation was then determined [78–80]. Ludmer et al. [11] found that injecting acetylcholine in normal coronary arteries produced endothelium-dependent vasodilatation, whereas in coronary arteries with moderate or severe atherosclerotic lesions a paradoxical vasoconstriction was obtained, indicating that endothelial dysfunction was present. The paradoxical vasoconstriction is due to stimulation of the muscarinic receptors of the smooth muscle cells by direct acetylcholine action. It was also found that injecting nitroglycerin, a NO donor, there was always vasodilatation, in this case considered as endothelium-independent vasodilatation. Vita et al. [81], using the same method, found that the amount of coronary vasodilatation obtained by acetylcholine diminished in an inverse ratio with the increase of total cholesterol or LDL-cholesterol levels. They also observed that the presence of cardiovascular risk factors, alone or combined, kept an inverse linear relationship with the endothelium-dependent vasodilator response, thus evidencing their additive effects on endothelial dysfunction [81].

Later, forearm plethysmography was used. This technique could be considered partially invasive. It was performed by placing the forearm in a plethysmograph for vein impedance and then injecting the study drug, usually acetylcholine or metacholine, into the brachial artery. Panza et al. [82–84], studying hypertensive patients, found them to have less vasodilator response than normal controls. Also, hypertensive patients had an increase in vascular resistance in comparison with normotensive individuals, which was permitted by endothelial dysfunction. As endothelium maintains a constant vasodilatation level produced by NO, it was considered that in hypertension there was an endothelial dysfunction that reduced NO release, and with that a reduced basal vasodilatation. This led them to postulate that endothelial dysfunction could be one of the causes of hypertension. Later on, other working groups concluded that endothelial dysfunction was probably a consequence and not the cause of hypertension [82–84]. This technique mainly evaluates the response of the resistance arteries.

In the last years, Celermajer et al. [85] assessed the level of vasodilatation by ultrasonography. This technique, noninvasive and easy to repeat, due to the changes that occur through time, allows us to learn the natural evolution of the disease or see the changes produced by the different treatments given. It consists of causing forearm ischemia and observes the amount of postischemic vasodilatation. Ischemia is produced by compressing the forearm by inflating a conventional cuff for measuring blood pressure 30 mm Hg above systolic pressure for 5 min. When pressure is released there is a marked increase in flow to the forearm and this increases shear stress, which in turn, stimulates NO release that causes vasodilatation. The amount of vasodilatation is directly proportional to the amount of NO released by the endothelium and this allows us to evaluate endothelial function. The increases in flow and vasodilatation are measured by high-resolution ultrasonography of the brachial artery, and are expressed as a percentage of basal values [85, 86]. The test can also be performed on the radial and femoral arteries [85, 87]. This technique evaluates mainly the conductance vessels, whereas plethysmography mainly evaluates resistance vessels, although both methods test NO release (fig. 4).

This method has shown a gradual decrease in the endothelium-dependent response depending on age, due to gradual loss of NO synthesis by the endothelial cells [88–90]. This same response is seen in patients with atherosclerotic lesions whether symptomatic or asymptomatic [90–92], in postmenopausal women due to the lack of estrogens [93, 94] and in presence of cardiovascular risk factors such as hypercholesterolemia [95], hypertension [96], active smoking [97, 98], passive smoking [99], obesity [100], diabetes [101], sedentary lifestyle [102] and hyperhomocysteinemia [103]. Mild infections [104] and increasing levels of CPR may also decrease the endothelial response [105]. Reversal of the cardiovascular risk factors allows a better endothelial function increasing endothelium-dependent vasodilatation which expresses an increase in NO release. Reduction of serum cholesterol levels [106–110], arterial pressure control [96, 106], quitting smoking [97], weight control [100], diabetes improvement [111], and physical activity [112] improve the endothelium-dependent response, indicating the release of more ON. The administration of L-arginine, an NO precursor, increases vasodilatation in patients with high cholesterol, coronary artery disease and heart failure [113–116]. As has been mentioned previously, all these risk factors act by a common pathway, oxidative stress, with increased production of ROS [117, 118]. It has been observed that giving antioxidant vitamins C and E diminishes the production of ROS [119–121], including when given before a meal with a high fat content to reduce oxidation of post absorption fatty acids and triglycerides [122]; this is also effective before smoking [123]. Recently, it has been reported that there is an additive effect with the simultaneous administration of a statin and

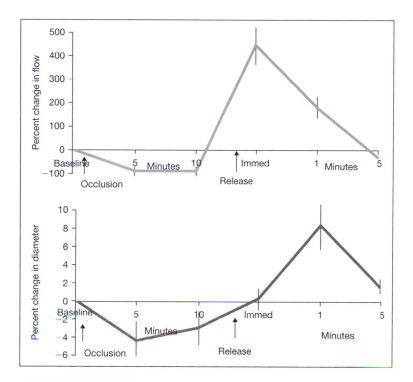

Fig. 4. Flow-mediated postischemic endothelial-dependent vasodilatation. Percent change in flow and diameter after occlusion. From Correti et al. [86].

an ACE inhibitor in hypercholesterolemic coronary artery disease patients (fig. 5) [124].

Although the method of evaluating endothelial responses by measurements on the brachial artery is noninvasive and easily repeated, without any risk to the patient, it is time consuming and needs skilled and patient operators [77, 125]. With just a small displacement of the transducer the results are altered. Some automated systems have shown a reduction in the variation between operators [77, 126, 127]. Some investigators have developed different equipment to maintain the transducer in a constant position. It is a well-known fact that the response is different according to whether the cuff is positioned on the arm or forearm. Recently, an International task force published the guidelines for the techniques and assessment of this method [87].

Looking for simpler methods for performing these procedures, laser-Doppler has recently been used. This technique considers the vasodilatation and the increase in blood flow, evaluating tissue perfusion. It has the advantage

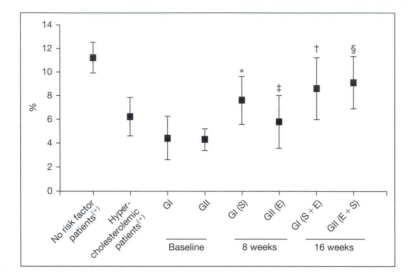

Fig. 5. Flow-mediated postischemic endothelium-dependent vasodilatation expressed as percent increase in arterial diameter (mean ± SD) with respect to baseline values in hypercholesterolemic coronary artery disease patients under the effects of the statin simvastatin and the ECA inhibitor enalapril, either separately or combined. E = Enalapril; GI = group I; GII = group II; S = simvastatin. *$p < 0.001$ vs. baseline, ‡$p < 0.01$ vs. baseline, †$p < 0.05$ vs. 8 weeks, §$p < 0.001$ vs. 8 weeks. From Esper et al. [124].

of being simple with immediate results and does not need skilled operators [128, 129].

Diabetes and Endothelium

Both type 1 (insulin-dependent) and type 2 (non-insulin-dependent) diabetic patients have mostly been described under enhanced oxidative stress, and both conditions are known to be powerful and independent risk factors for coronary heart disease, stroke, and peripheral arterial disease.

Hyperglycemia causes glycosylation of proteins and phospholipids, thus increasing intracellular oxidative stress. Nonenzymatic reactive products, known as Maillard or browning reaction, glucose-derived Schiff base, and Amadori products, form chemically reversible early glycosylation products which subsequently rearrange to form more stable products, some of them long-lived proteins (e.g. vessel wall collagen), which continue undergoing a complex series of chemical rearrangements to form advanced glycosylation

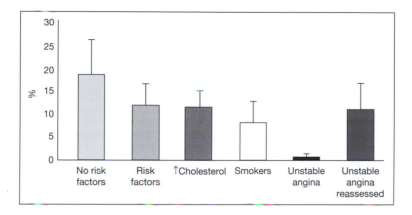

Fig. 6. Endothelium-dependent vasodilatation in subjects with no cardiovascular risk factors and in patients with risk factors (hypercholesterolemic and smokers) within 24 h of rapidly stabilized unstable angina, and approximately 30 days later, after pharmacological treatment. From Esper et al. [132].

end-products (AGEs). Once formed, AGEs are stable and virtually irreversible. AGEs generate ROS with consequent increased vessel oxidative damage [130].

Phagocytes have specialized receptors for AGEs, their activation leading to oxidation of lipoproteins, especially the phospholipid component in LDL, thus triggering an immuno-inflammatory response and a thrombogenic response through tromboxane A_2 release and platelet aggregation induction. Diabetic patients have increased levels of inflammatory markers, including CRP, with pro-inflammatory and pro-atherogenic properties.

The impressive correlation between coronary artery disease and alterations in glucose metabolism has raised the hypothesis that atherosclerosis and diabetes may share common antecedents. Large-vessel atherosclerosis can precede the development of diabetes, suggesting that rather than atherosclerosis being a complication of diabetes, both conditions may share genetic and environmental antecedents, a 'common soil' [131].

Our group [132] found that endothelium-dependent vasodilatation during unstable angina is practically absent, creating a doubt about whether 'the endothelial dysfunction is caused by the plaque rupture or if it existed previously and did not protect the high-risk atheromatous plaque allowing the acute coronary event'. Based on this study and comparing with what happens to the ischemic myocardium created the concept of 'stunned' endothelium to explain the low vasodilatation response in acute ischemia and 'hibernated' endothelium when a poor response is chronic, as observed with hypercholesterolemia and the presence of other risk factors (fig. 6).

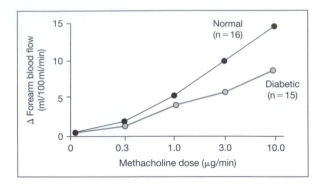

Fig. 7. Impaired flow-mediated endothelial-dependent vasodilation in diabetic patients. Adapted from Johnstone et al. [101].

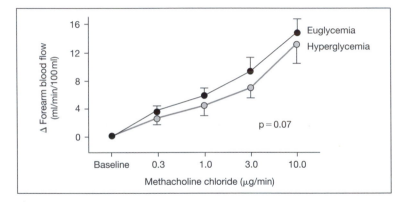

Fig. 8. Impaired blood flow-mediated endothelial-dependent vasodilation in normal individuals with induced hyperglycemia. Adapted from Williams et al. [133].

Published data suggest that abnormal endothelial function precedes other evidence of vascular disease and that the progression of metabolic syndrome to type 2 diabetes parallels the progression of endothelial dysfunction to atherosclerosis (fig. 7) [101]. Both type 1 and type 2 diabetes, like metabolic syndrome and other cardiovascular risk factors, determine an abnormal endothelium response thought to precede the development of atherosclerosis. A transient rise in glycemia has been shown to be enough to cause endothelial dysfunction (fig. 8) [133].

All of these assumptions lead to the hypothesis that patients with either metabolic syndrome or type 1 or 2 diabetes may have a reduced bioavailability of NO or a lessened response to it by the smooth muscle cell of the vascular wall. Besides, it has been noticed that the presence of diabetes abolishes differences in mortality between genders by enhancing it in women, though it is not possible to rule out an impaired glycemic control with greater levels of glycosylated hemoglobin A1c or a diminished compliance with treatment, conditions frequently seen in women [134].

Studies in animal models have always shown that endothelial dysfunction is present in diabetic individuals though in humans dissimilar responses have been observed [135]. However, in any circumstances an impaired vasodilator response to nitrites has been detected, allowing for the assumption of a diminished response to NO by the smooth muscle cell of the arterial wall, though in some studies differences were not statistically significant [136]. These facts could account for the improvement observed in diabetic individuals treated with ACE inhibitors or AT1 receptor blockers, whose activation antagonize the effects of NO [137].

The magnitude of endothelial dysfunction in diabetics is often related to the severity and duration of the illness, as well as to glycemic and glycosylated hemoglobin A1c levels, and to the lack of adherence to treatment, this being so important as to overshadow the actions of the other risk factors. However, it has been observed that diabetics who have been treated with statins to reduce cholesterol levels, or have quit smoking and increased their physical activities, achieved greater improvements in endothelial function than those who were only subjected to the treatment of hyperglycemia, which is in agreement with the current guidelines for the treatment of diabetes [138].

References

1   Rubanyi GM: The role of endothelium in cardiovascular homeostasis and diseases. J Cardiovasc Pharmacol 1993;22(suppl 4):S1–S14.
2   Drenckham D, Ness W: The endothelial contractile cytoskeleton; in Born GVR, Schwartz CJ (eds): Vascular Endothelium: Physiology, Pathology, and Therapeutic Opportunities. Stuttgart, Schattauer, 1997, pp 1–25.
3   Andersen RGW: Caveolae: where incoming and outgoing messengers meet. Proc Natl Acad Sci USA 1993;90:10909–10913.
4   Esper RJ, Vilariño JO: La disfunción endotelial. Consideraciones fisiopatológicas y diagnósticas; en Esper RJ, Vilariño JO (eds): La placa de alto riesgo. Barcelona, Prous Sciences, 2002, pp 19–43.
5   Esper RJ, Vilariño JO: La disfunción endotelial; en Esper RJ (ed): Aterotrombosis en el tercer milenio. Barcelona, Prous Sciences, 2004, pp 49–83.
6   Vanhoutte PM: How to assess endothelial function in human blood vessels. J Hypertens 1999;17: 1047–1058.
7   Loscalzo J, Welch G: Nitric oxide and its role in the cardiovascular system. Prog Cardiovasc Dis 1995;38:87–104.
8   Jones CJH, Kuo L, Davis MJ, deFily DV, Chillian WM: Role of nitric oxide in coronary microvascular responses to adenosine and increased metabolic demand. Circulation 1996;91:1807–1813.

9 Cooke JP, Tsao PS: Go with the flow. Circulation 2001;103:2773–2775.

10 Miura H, Watchel RE, Liu Y, Loberiza F, Saito T, Miura M, Gutterman DD: Flow-induced dilation of human coronary arterioles: important role of Ca(2+)-activated K(+) channels. Circulation 2001;103:1992–1998.

11 Ludmer PL, Selwyn AP, Shook TL, Wayne RR, Mufge GH, Alexander RW, Ganz P: Paradoxical vasoconstriction induced by acetylcholine in atherosclerosis coronary arteries. N Engl J Med 1986;315:1046–1051.

12 Asakura K, Karino T: Flow patterns and spatial distribution of atherosclerosis lesions in human coronary arteries. Circ Res 1990;66:1045–1066.

13 Makek AM, Alper SL, Izumo S: Hemodynamic shear stress and its role in atherosclerosis. JAMA 1999;282:2035–2042.

14 Jalali S, Li YS, Sotoudeh M, Yuan S, Li S, Chien S, Shyy JY: Shear stress activates p60src-Ras-MAPK signaling pathways in vascular endothelial cells. Arterioscler Thromb Vasc Biol 1998;18:227–234.

15 Feldman CL, Stone PH: Intravascular hemodynamic factors responsible for progression of coronary atherosclerosis and development of vulnerable plaque. Curr Opin in Cardiol 2000;15:430–440.

16 Cooke JP, Tsao PS: Is NO an endogenous antiatherogenic molecule?. Arterioscler Thromb 1994;14:753–759.

17 Baldwin A: The transcription factor NK-6B and human disease. J Clin Invest 2001;107:3–6.

18 Tak P, Firestein G: NF-6B: a key role in inflammatory disease. J Clin Invest 2001;107:7–11.

19 Libby P: Current concepts of the pathogenesis of the acute coronary syndrome. Circulation 2001;104:365–372.

20 Thurberg B, Collins T: The nuclear factor-kappa B/inhibitor of kappa B autoregulatory system and atherosclerosis. Curr Opin Lipidol 1998;9:387–396.

21 Marx N, Sukhova GK, Collins T: PPARα activactors inhibitor cytokine-induced vascular cell adhesion molecule-1 expression in human endothelial cells. Circulation 1999;99:3125–3131.

22 Marx N, Mackman N, Schoenbeck U: PPARα activactors inhibit tissue factor expression and activity in human monocytes. Circulation 2001;103:213–219.

23 Dzau VJ: Vascular angiotensin pathways: a new therapeutic target. J Cardiovasc Pharmacol 1987;10(suppl 7):S9–S16.

24 Johnston CJ: Renin-angiotensin system: a dual tissue and hormonal system for cardiovascular control. J Cardiovasc Pharmacol 1992;20(suppl B):S1–S5.

25 Kawano H, Do YS, Kawano Y, Starnes V, Barr M, Law RE, Hsueh WA: Angiotensin II has multiple profibrotic effects in human cardiac fibroblast. Circulation 2000;101:1130–1137.

26 Biasucci LM, Vitelli A, Liuzzo G, Altamura S, Caliguri G, Monaco C, Rabuzzi AG, Ciliberto G, Maseri A: Elevated levels of interleukin-6 in unstable angina. Circulation 1996;94:874–877.

27 Kacimi R, Long CS, Karliner JS: Chronic hypoxia modulates the interleukin-1β-stimulated inducible nitric oxide synthase pathway in cardiac myocytes. Circulation 1997;96:1937–1943.

28 Torre-Amione G, Kapadia S, Lee J, Bies RD, Lebovitz R, Mann DL: Expression and functional significance of tumor necrosis factor receptors in human myocardium. Circulation 1995;92:1487–1493.

29 Smith SC, Allen PM: Neutralization of endogenous tumor necrosis factor ameliorates the severity of myosin-induced myocarditis. Circ Res 1992;70:856–863.

30 Matsumori A, Yamada T, Suzuki H, Matoba Y, Sasayama S: Increased circulating cytokines in patients with myocarditis and cardiomyopathy. Br Heart J 1994;72:561–566.

31 Valen G, Yan Z, Hansson GK: Nuclear factor Kappa-B and the heart. J Am Coll Cardiol 2001;38:307–314.

32 Siragy H: Angiotensin II receptor blockers: review of the binding characteristics. Am J Cardiol 1999;84(suppl):3–8.

33 Nickening G, Harrison DG: The AT1-type angiotensin receptor in oxidative stress and atherogenesis. I. Oxidative stress and atherogenesis. Circulation 2002;105:393–396.

34 Benter IF, Ferrario CM, Morris M, Diz DI: Antihypertensive actions of angiotensin(1–7) in spontaneously hypertensive rats. Am J Physiol 1995;269:H313–H319.

35 Givertz MM, Sawyer DB, Colucci WS: Antioxidants and myocardial contractility: illuminating the 'dark side' of β-adrenergic receptor activation. Circulation 2001;103:782–783.

36 Peiser L, Mukhopadhyay S, Gordon S: Scavenger receptors in innate immunity. Curr Opin Immunol 2002;14:123–128.

37 Janeway CA Jr, Medzhitov R: Innate immune recognition. Annu Rev Immunol 2002;20:197–216.

38 Leitinger N: Oxidized phospholipids as modulators of inflammation in atherosclerosis. Curr Opin Lipid 2003;14:421–430.

39 Li D, Mehta JL: Antisense to LOX-1 inhibits oxidized LDL-mediated up-regulation of monocyte chemoatractant protein-1 and monocyte adhesion to human coronary artery endothelial cells. Circulation 2000;101:2889–2895.

40 Tsimikas S, Witztum JL: Measuring circulating oxidized low-density lipoprotein to evaluate coronary risk. Circulation 2001;103:1930–1932.

41 Libby P: Molecular bases of the acute coronary syndromes. Circulation 1995;91:2844–2850.

42 Li D, Mehta JL: Up-regulation of endothelial receptor for oxidized LDL (LOX 1) by oxidized and implications in apoptosis of human coronary artery endothelial cells: evidence from use of antisense LOX-1 mRNA and chemical inhibitors. Ateroscler Thromb Vasc Biol 2000;20: 1116–1122.

43 Kadokami T, Frye C, Lemster B, Wagner CL, Feldman AM, McTiernan CF: Anti-Tumor necrosis factor-α antibody limits heart failure in a transgenic model. Circulation 2001;104:1094–1097.

44 Shah P, Kaul S, Nilsson J, Cercek B: Exploiting the vascular protective effects of high-density lipoprotein and its apolipoproteins: an idea whose time for testing is coming. Part I. Circulation 2001;104:2376–2383.

45 Böger R, Bode-Böger S, Szuba A, Tsao PS, Chan JR, Tangphao O, Blaschke TF, Cooke JP: Asymmetric dimethylarginine (ADMA): a novel risk factor for endothelial dysfunction. Circulation 1998;98:1842–1847.

46 Ehara S, Ueda M, Naruko T, Haze K: Elevated levels of oxidated low density lipoprotein show a positive relationship with the severity of acute coronary syndrome. Circulation 2001;103: 1955–1960.

47 Landmesser U, Harrison DG: Oxidant stress and marker for cardiovascular events. Ox marks the spots. Circulation 2001;104:2638–2640.

48 Sage PR, de la Lande IS, Stafford I, Bennett CL, Phillipov G, Stubberfield J, Horowitz JD: Nitroglycerin tolerance in human vessels: evidence for impaired nitroglycerin bioconversion. Circulation 2000;102:2810–2815.

49 Gori T, Burstein JM, Ahmed S, Miner SES, Al-Hesayen A, Kelly S, Parker JD: Folic acid prevents nitroglycerin-induced nitric oxide synthase dysfunction and nitrate tolerance: a human in vivo study. Circulation 2001;104:1119–1123.

50 March F, Schoembeck U, Bonnefoy JY: Activation of the monocyte/macrophage related to acute atheroma complication by ligation of CD-40 induction of collagenase, stromelysin, and tissue factor. Circulation 1997;96:396–399.

51 Henn V, Slupsky JR, Grafe M: CD-40 ligand on activated platelets triggers an inflammatory reaction of endothelial cells. Nature 1998;391:591–594.

52 von Hundelshausen P, Weber KSC, Huo Y: RANTES deposition by platelets triggers monocyte arrest on inflamed and atherosclerotic endothelium. Circulation 2001;103:1772–1777.

53 Yeh ETH, Anderson V, Pasceri V, Willerson JT: C-reactive protein: linking inflammation to cardiovascular complications. Circulation 2001;104:974–975.

54 Fuster V, Moreno P, Fayad ZA, Corti R, Badimon JJ: Atherothrombosis and high-risk plaque. I. Evolving concepts. J Am Coll Cardiol 2005;46:937–954.

55 Libby P, Simon DI: Inflammation and trombosis: the clot thickens. Circulation 2001;103: 1718–1720.

56 Nicoletti A, Caliguri G, Paulosson G: Functionality of specific immunity in atherosclerosis. Am Heart J 1999;138:438–443.

57 Mackay IR, Rosen FS: Autoimmune disease. N Engl J Med 2001;345:340–350.

58 Mosmann Tr, Cherwinsky H, Bond MW: Two type of murine helper-T cell clone: definition according to profiles of lymphokine activities and secreted proteins. J Immunol 1986;136:2348–2357.

59 Lee TS, Yen HC, Pann CC: The role of interleukin 12 in the development of the atherosclerosis in apo E-deficient mice. Atherioscler Thromb Vasc Biol 1999;19:734–742.
60 Zhou X, Paulsson G, Stemme S: Hypercholesterolemia is associated with a T-helper Th1/Th2 switch of the immune response in apo E-knockout mice. J Clin Invest 1998;101:1717–1725.
61 Pasceri V, Yeh ET: A tale of two diseases: atherosclerosis and rheumatoid arthritis. Circulation 1999;100:2124–2126.
62 Laurat E, Poirier B, Tupin E: In vivo downregulation of T-helper cell 1 immune responses reduces atherosclerosis in apolipoprotein E-knockout mice. Circulation 2001;104:197–202.
63 Kak B, Mulhaupt F, Myit S: Statins as newly recognized type of immunomodulator. Nat Med 2000;6:1399–1402.
64 Palinsky W: Immunomodulation: a new role for statins? Nat Med 2000;6:1311–1312.
65 Hansson GK: Inflammation, atherosclerosis, and coronary artery disease. N Engl J Med 2005;352: 1685–1695.
66 Wong ML, Xie B, Beatini N, Phu P: Acute systemic inflammation up-regulates secretory sphingomyelinase in vivo: a possible link between inflammatory cytokines and atherosclerosis. PNAS 2000;97:8681–8686.
67 Xian CJ, Paultre F, Pearson TA, Reed RG: Plasma sphingomyelin level as a Risk Factor for coronary artery disease. Arterioscler Throm Vasc Biol 2000;20:2614–2618.
68 Hansson GK: Inflammation, atherosclerosis, and coronary artery disease. N Engl J Med 2005;352: 1685–1695.
69 Falk E, Shah PK, Fuster V: Coronary plaque disruption. Circulation 1995;92:657–671.
70 Ziada KM, Vince DG, Nissen SE, Tuzcu EM: Arterial remodeling and coronary artery disease: the concept of 'dilated' versus 'obstructive' coronary atherosclerosis. J Am Coll Cardiol 2001;38: 297–306.
71 Ross R: Atherosclerosis: an inflammatory disease. N Engl J Med 1999;340:115–126.
72 Danesch J, Whincup P, Walker M, Lennon L, Thomson A, Appleby P, Rumley A, Lowe GDO: Fibrin D-dimer and coronary heart disease: prospective study and meta-analysis. Circulation 2001;103:2323–2327.
73 Manunucci M: Von Willebrand factor: a marker of endothelial damage. Atheroscler Thromb Vasc Biol 1998;18:1359–1362.
74 Thompson SG, Kienast J, Pyke SD, Haverkate F: Hemostatic factors and the risk of myocardial infarction and sudden death in patients with angina pectoris. N Engl J Med 1995;332: 635–641.
75 Jensen JS, Feldt-Rasmussen BF, Strandgaard S, Schroll M, Borch-Johnson K: Hypertension, microalbuminuria and risk of cardiac ischemic disease. Hypertension 2000;35:898–903.
76 Fuster V: Remodelado del trombo: un punto clave en la progresión de la aterosclerosis coronaria. Rev Española Cardiol 2000;53(suppl 11):2–7.
77 Esper RJ: Interrogando al endotelio. Rev Argent Cardiol 2000;68:429–439.
78 Esper RJ: Detección de la placa de alto riesgo. Intercontinent Cardiol 2001;10:63–70.
79 Fisman E, Esper RJ, Tenenbaum A: Diabetes y Enfermedad Cardiovascular: Aspectos Fisiopatológicos y Clínicos del Síndrome Metabólico y la Insuficiencia Cardíaca Congestiva. Buenos Aires, Maestría en Ateroesclerosis, 2005, vol 8, pp 1–32.
80 Vilariño JO, Esper RJ, Badimon JJ: Fisopatología de los Síndromes Coronarios Agudos. Tres paradigmas para un solo dogma. Rev Española Cardiol 2004;4(suppl G):13G–24G.
81 Vita JA, Treasure CB, Nabel EG: Coronary vasomotor response to acetylcholine relate to risk factor for coronary artery disease. Circulation 1990;81:491–498.
82 Panza JA, Quyyumi AA, Brush JE Jr, Epstein SE: Abnormal endothelium-dependent vascular relaxation in patients with essential hypertension. N Engl J Med 1990;323:22–27.
83 Panza JA, Casino PR, Kilcoyne CM, Quyyumi AA: Role of the endothelium-derived nitric oxide in the abnormal endothelium-dependent vascular relaxation in patients with essential hypertension. Circulation 1993;87:1468–1474.
84 Panza JA, Quyyumi AA, Callahan TS, Epstein SE: Effect of antihypertensive treatment of endothelium-dependent vascular relaxation in patients with essential hypertension. J Am Coll Cardiol 1993;21:1145–1151.
85 Celermajer DS, Sorensen KE, Gooch VM, Spiegelhalter DJ, Miller OI, Sullivan ID, Lloyd JK, Deanfield JE: Non-invasive detection of endothelial dysfunction in children and adults at risk of atherosclerosis. Lancet 1992;340:1111–1115.

86 Corretti MC, Plotnik GD, Vogel RA: Technical aspects of evaluating brachial artery vasodilatation using high-frequency ultrasound. Am J Physiol 1995;268:H1397–H1404.

87 Corretti MC, Todd J, Anderson TJ, Benjamin EJ, Celermajer DS, Charbonneau F, Creager MA, Deanfield JE, Drexler H, Gerhard-Herman M, Herrington D, Vallance P, Vita J, Vogel R: Guidelines for the ultrasound assessment of endotelial-dependent flow-mediated vasodilation of the brachial artery. J Am Coll Cardiol 2002;39:257–265.

88 Zeiher AM, Drexler H, Saurier B, Just H: Endothelium-mediated coronary blood flow modulation in humans: effect of age, atherosclerosis, hypercholesterolemia, and hypertension. J Clin Invest 1993;92:652–662.

89 Celermajer DS, Sorensen KE, Spiegelhalter DJ, Georgakopoulos D, Robinson J, Deanfield JE: Ageing is associated with endothelial dysfunction in healthy men years before the age-related decline in women. J Am Coll Cardiol 1994;24:471–476.

90 Vilariño JO, Cacharrón JL, Suarez DH, Kura M, Machado R, Bolaño AL, Esper RJ: Evaluación de la función endotelial por eco-Doppler. Influencia de la edad, sexo y factores de riesgo. Rev Argent Cardiol 1998;66:523–532.

91 Gordon JB, Ganz P, Nabel EG, Fish RD, Zebede J, Mudge GH, Alexander RW, Selwyn AP: Atherosclerosis influence the vasomotor response of epicardial coronary arteries to exercise. J Clin Invest 1989;83:1946–1952.

92 Nabel EG, Selwyn AP, Ganz P: Large coronary arteries in humans are responsive to changing blood flow: an endothelium-dependent mechanism that fail in patients with atherosclerosis. J Am Coll Cardiol 1990;16:349–356.

93 Williams JK, Adams MR, Klopfenstein HS: Estrogen modulates responses of atherosclerotic coronary arteries. Circulation 1990;81:1680–1687.

94 Lieberman EH, Gerhard MD, Uehata A, Walsh BW, Selwyn AP, Ganz P, Yeung AC, Creager MA: Estrogen improves endothelium-dependent, flow-mediated vasodilation in postmenopausal women. Ann Intern Med 1994;121:936–941.

95 Creager MA, Cooke JP, Mendelsohn ME, Gallagher SJ, Coleman SM, Loscalzo J, Dzau VJ: Impaired vasodilatation of forearm resistance vessels in hypercholesterolemic humans. J Clin Invest 1990;86:228–234.

96 Panza JA, Cannon RO III (eds): Endothelium, Nitric Oxide, and Atherosclerosis. New York, Futura Publishing, 1999.

97 Celermajer DS, Sorensen KE, Georgakopoulos D, Bull C, Tomas O, Robinson J, Deanfield JE: Cigarette smoking is associated with dose-related and potentially reversible impairment of endothelium-dependent dilation in healthy young adults. Circulation 1993;88:2149–2155.

98 Zeiher A, Schächinger V, Minners J: Long-term cigarette smoking impairs endothelium-dependent coronary vasodilator function. Circulation 1995;92:1094–1100.

99 Celermajer DS, Adams MR, Clarkson P, Robinson J, McCredie R, Donald A, Denfield JE: Passive smoking and impaired endothelium-dependent arterial dilatation in healthy young adults. N Engl J Med 1996;334:150–154.

100 Mark AL, Correia M, Morgan DA, Schaffer RA, Haynes WG: Obesity-induced hypertension: new concepts from de emerging biology of obesity. Hypertension 1999;33:537–541.

101 Johnstone MT, Creager SJ, Scales KM, Cusko JA, Lee BK, Creager MA: Impaired endothelium-dependent vasodilation in patients with insulin-dependent diabetes mellitus. Circulation 1993;88:2510–2516.

102 Snell PG, Mitchell JH: Physical inactivity: an easily modified risk factor?. Circulation 1999;100:2–4.

103 Celermajer DS, Sorensen K, Ryalls M, Robinson J, Thomas O, Leonard JV, Deanfield JE: Impaired endothelial function occurs in the systemic arteries of children with homozygous homo-cystinuria but not in their heterozygous parents. J Am Coll Cardiol 1993;22:854–858.

104 Charakida M., Donald AE, Terese M, Leary S, Halcox JP, Ness A, Smith GD, Golding J, Friberg P, Klein NJ, Deanfield JE: Endothelial dysfunction in childhood infection. Circulation 2005;111:1660–1665.

105 Fichtlscherer S, Rosenberg G, Walter DH, Breuer S, Dimmeler S, Zehier AM: Elevated C Reactive Protein levels impaired endothelial vasoreactivity in patients with coronary artery disease. Circulation 2000;102:1000–1006.

106 Egashira K, Hirooka Y, Kai H, Sugimachi M, Suzuki S, Inou T, Takeshita A: Reduction in serum cholesterol with pravastatin improves endothelium-dependent vasomotion in patients with hypercholesterolemia. Circulation 1994;89:2519–2524.

107 Treasure CB, Klein JL, Weintraub WS, Talley JD, Stillabouer ME, Kosinski AS, Zhang J, Bocuzzi SJ, Cedarholm JC, Alexander RW: Beneficial effects of cholesterol-lowering therapy on the coronary endothelium in patients with coronary artery disease. N Engl J Med 1995;332:481–487.

108 Waters D: Cholesterol lowering: should it continue to be the last thing we do. Circulation 1999;99: 3215–3217.

109 Esper RJ: The role of lipid-lowering therapy in multiple risk factor management. Drugs 1998;56(suppl 1):1–7.

110 Webb D, Vallance P (eds): Endothelial Function in Hypertension. Berlin, Springer, 1997.

111 Murakami T, Mizuno S, Ohsato K, Moriuchi I, Arai Y, Nio Y, Kaku B, Takahashi Y, Ohnaka M: Effects of troglitazone on frequency of coronary vasospastic-induced angina pectoris in patients with diabetes mellitus. Am J Cardiol 1999;84:92–94.

112 Horning B, Maier V, Drexler H: Physical training improves endothelial function in patients with chronic heart failure. Circulation 1996;93:210–214.

113 Creager MA, Gallagher SJ, Girerd XJ, Coleman SM, Dzau VJ, Cooke JP: L-Arginine improves endothelium-dependent vasodilation in hypercholesterolemic humans. J Clin Invest 1992;90: 1248–1253.

114 Drexler H, Zeiher AM, Meinertz T, Just H: Correcting endothelial dysfunction in coronary microcirculation of hypercholesterolemic patients by L-arginine. Lancet 1991;338:1546–1550.

115 Clarkson D, Adams MR, Powe A, et al: Oral L-arginine improves endothelium-dependent dilation in hypercholesterolemic young adults. J Clin Invest 1996;97:1989–1994.

116 Griendling KK, FitzGerald GA: Oxidative stress and cardiovascular injury. I. Basic mechanisms and in vivo monitoring of ROS. Circulation 2003;108:1912–1916.

117 Ridker PM, Cushman M, Stampfer MJ, Tracy RP, Hennekens CH: Inflammation, aspirin and the risk of cardiovascular disease in apparently healthy men. N Engl J Med 1997;336:973–979.

118 Ridker PM: Inflammation, infection and cardiovascular risk: how good is the clinical evidence? Circulation 1998;96:1671–1674.

119 Levine GN, Frei B, Koulouris SN, Gerhard MD, Keaney JF, Vita JA: Ascorbic acid reverses endothelial vasomotor dysfunction in patients with coronary artery disease. Circulation 1996;93: 1107–1113.

120 Gokce N, Keaney JF Jr, Frei B, et al: Long-term ascorbic acid administration reverses endothelial vasomotor dysfunction in patients with coronary artery disease. Circulation 1999;99:3234–3240.

121 Solzbach U, Hornig B, Jeserich M, Hanjörg J: Vitamin C improves endothelial dysfunction of epicardial coronary arteries in hypertensive patients. Circulation 1997;96:1513–1519.

122 Plotnick GD, Corretti MC, Vogel RA: Effect of antioxidant vitamins on the transient impairment of endothelial-dependent brachial artery vasoactivity following a single high-fat meal. JAMA 1997;278:1682–1686.

123 Heitzer T, Just H, Munzel T: Antioxidant vitamin C improves endothelial dysfunction in chronic smokers. Circulation 1996;94:6–9.

124 Esper RJ, Machado R, Vilariño J, Cacharrón JL, Ingino CA, García Guiñazú CA, Bereziuk E, Bolaño LA, Suarez DH: Endothelium-dependent response in hypercholesterolemic coronary artery disease patients under the effects of simvastatin and enalapril, either separately o combined. Am Heart J 2000;140:684–689.

125 Esper RJ, Nordaby RA, Vilariño JO, Paragano A, Cacharrón JL, Machado RA: Endothelial dysfunction: a comprehensive appraisal. Cardiovasc Diabetol 2006;5:4.

126 Hijmering ML, Stroes ES, Pasterkamp G: Variability of flow mediated dilation: consequences for clinical application. Atherosclerosis 2001;157:369–373.

127 Kuvin JT, Patel AR, Karas RH: Need for standardization of noninvasive assessment of vascular endothelial function. Am Heart J 2001;141:327–328.

128 Pergola PE, Kellogg DL, Johnson JM, Kosiba WA, Salomon DE: Role of the sympathetic nerves in the vascular effects of local temperature in human forearm skin. Am J Physiol 1993;265: H785–H792.

129 Rauch U, Osende JI, Chesebro JH, Badimon JJ: Statins and cardiovascular diseases: the multiple effects of lipid-lowering therapy by statins. Atherosclerosis 2000;153:181–189.

130 Stern MP: Diabetes and cardiovascular disease: the 'common soil' hypothesis. Diabetes 1995; 44:369–374.

131 Tselepis AD, John CM: Inflammation, bioactive lipids and atherosclerosis: potential roles of a lipoprotein-associated phospholipase A2, platelet activating factor-acetylhydrolase. Atherosclerosis 2002;3(suppl):57–68.

132 Esper RJ, Vilariño J, Cacharrón JL, Machado R, Ingino CA, García Guiñazú CA, Bereziuk E, Bolaño AL, Suarez DH, Kura M: Impaired endothelial function in patients with rapidly stabilized unstable angina: assessment by noninvasive brachial artery ultrasonography. Clin Cardiol 1999;22:699–703.

133 Williams SB, Goldfine AB, Timimi FK, Ting HH, Roddy MA, Simonson DC, Creager MA: Acute hyperglycemia attenuates endothelium-dependent vasodilation in humans in vivo. Circulation 1998;97:1695–1701.

134 Chan NN, Vallance P, Colhoun HM: Endothelium-dependent and -independent vascular dysfunction in type 1 diabetes. Arterioscler Thromb Vasc Biol 2003;23:1048–1054.

135 De Vriese AC, Verbeuren TJ, Van D, Lameire NH, Vanhoutte PM: Endothelial dysfunction in diabetes. Br J Pharmacol 2000;130:963–974.

136 Smits P, Kapma JA, Jacobs MC, Lutterman J, Thien T: Endothelium-dependent vascular relaxation in patients with type 1 diabetes. Diabetes 1993;42:148–153.

137 Clarkson P, Celermajer DS, Donald AE, Sampson M, Sorensen KE, Adams M, et al: Impaired vascular reactivity in insulin-dependent diabetes mellitus is related to disease duration and low density lipoprotein cholesterol levels. Am J Coll Cardiol 1996;28:573–579.

138 Koivisto VA, Stevens LK, Mattock M, Ebeling P, Muggeo M, Stephenson J, Idzior-Walus B: The EURODIAB IDDM complications study group: cardiovascular disease and its risk factors in IDDM in Europe. Diabetes Care 1996;19:689–697.

Prof. Ricardo J. Esper
University del Salvador
Virrey Loreto 2111
C1426DXM Buenos Aires (Argentina)
E-Mail ricardo.esper@fibertel.com.ar

Fisman EZ, Tenenbaum A (eds): Cardiovascular Diabetology: Clinical, Metabolic and Inflammatory
Facets. Adv Cardiol. Basel, Karger, 2008, vol 45, pp 44–64

....

Biomarkers in Cardiovascular Diabetology: Interleukins and Matrixins

Enrique Z. Fisman[a]   *Yehuda Adler*[b]   *Alexander Tenenbaum*[a,b]

[a] Cardiovascular Diabetology Research Foundation, Holon, [b] Cardiac Rehabilitation
Institute, Chaim Sheba Medical Center, Tel-Hashomer, affiliated to the Sackler Faculty
of Medicine, Tel-Aviv University, Tel-Aviv, Israel

Abstract

The impressive correlation between cardiovascular disease and alterations in glucose
metabolism has raised the likelihood that atherosclerosis and type 2 diabetes may share common
antecedents. Inflammation is emerging as a conceivable etiologic mechanism for both.
Interleukins are regulatory proteins with ability to accelerate or inhibit inflammatory processes,
and matrixins are prepro enzymes responsible for the timely breakdown of extracellular matrix.
Interleukins (ILs) are classified based on their role in diabetes and atherosclerosis, hypothesizing
that each interleukin acts on both diseases in the same direction – regardless if harmful, favorable or neutral. They are clustered into three groups: noxious (the 'bad', 8 members), comprising
IL-1, IL-2, IL-6, IL-7, IL-8, IL-15, IL-17 and IL-18; protective (the 'good', 5 members), comprising IL-4, IL-10, IL-11, IL-12 and IL-13; and 'aloof' , comprising IL-5, IL-9, IL-14, IL-16
and IL-19 through IL-29 (15 members). Each group presented converging effects on both diseases. IL-3 was reluctant to clustering and IL-30 through 33 were not included due to the scarce
available data. It may be seen that (1) favorable effects of a given interleukin on either diabetes
or atherosclerosis predicts similar effects on the other; (2) equally, harmful interleukin effects on
one disease can be extrapolated to the other, and (3) absence of influence of a given interleukin on
one of these diseases forecasts lack of effects on the other. Matrixins seem to present a similar
pathophysiological pattern. These facts further support the unifying etiologic theory of diabetes
and heart disease, emphasizing the importance of a cardiovascular diabetologic approach to these
cytokines for future research. A pharmacologic simultaneous targeting of interleukins and matrixins might provide an effective means to concurrently control both atherosclerosis and diabetes.

Copyright © 2008 S. Karger AG, Basel

Background

The impressive correlation between coronary artery disease (CAD) and
alterations in glucose metabolism has raised the likelihood that atherosclerosis

and type 2 diabetes may share common antecedents. It is now known that adverse environmental conditions – perhaps related to less-than-optimal nutrition – in fetal and early life are associated with an enhanced risk of both diabetes and cardiovascular disease many decades later. Large-vessel atherosclerosis can precede the development of diabetes, suggesting that rather than atherosclerosis being a complication of diabetes, both conditions may share genetic and environmental antecedents, a 'common soil' [1]. These same adverse environmental conditions associated with hyperinsulinemia and insulin resistance lead to the development in adult life of the dysmetabolic syndrome, consisting of abdominal obesity, impaired fasting glucose, high triglyceride levels, low high-density lipoprotein levels and hypertension. These constituents may be associated with additional elements, such as elevations in small low-density lipoproteins, prothrombotic factors and free fatty acids [2]. Taking into consideration that the components of this cluster of abnormalities are essentially shared by both diabetes type 2 and atherosclerosis, the American Heart Association stated in 1999 that 'diabetes *is* a cardiovascular disease' [3]. Although the mechanism underlying this cluster is not yet fully clarified, the statistical association is well established [1].

In this context, chronic low-grade inflammation is emerging as a conceivable etiologic mechanism. Inflammation plays an important role in mediating all phases of atherosclerosis, from initial recruitment of circulating cells to the inner arterial layer to weakening of the fibrous cap of the plaque, eventually leading to rupture. Inflammation is heavily involved in the onset and development of atherothrombotic disease, which is accompanied by the emergence of numerous inflammatory biomarkers. Such biomarkers comprise a vast array of substances, including cytokines as the interleukins, matrixins, acute-phase proteins, adhesion molecules, tumor necrosis factor (TNF) and monocyte chemoattractant protein (MCP) isoforms, interferons, chemokines, etc. [4]. Several studies have demonstrated an association between these biomarkers and current or future overt CAD [5–7]. A close relation is also present between the biomarkers and glucose metabolism abnormalities. For instance, obese patients with impaired fasting glucose exhibit elevated concentrations of interleukin (IL)-8 [8], glucose increases monocyte adhesion to human aortic endothelial cells via stimulation of IL-8 [9], and elevated levels of IL-18 and TNF-α were found in serum of patients with type 2 diabetes mellitus [10]. Thus, a common inflammatory basis for both diabetes and CAD seems plausible [11].

Interleukins

Interleukins are probably the most extensively produced biomarkers. Considerable confusion exists regarding their clinical value, due to several factors: (1) increased levels of a given IL, presenting statistical correlation with disease, does not necessarily imply causation; (2) these compounds are characterized by substantial redundancy in that different interleukins have similar functions; (3) many of them are pleiotropic, with capability of acting on different cell types; (4) interleukins may stimulate secretion of other interleukins, enhancing or inhibiting each other; (5) interleukins possess 'paradoxical' effects, expressed as protective properties regarding a given system, whereas they may damage another system, and (6) protective or noxious effects of a given interleukin may be concentration-dependent.

A huge quantity of data regarding interleukins has been accumulating during the last two decades; a considerable part is dedicated to their effects on diabetes and cardiovascular function. However, no attempts have been made to present a systematic classification of interleukins based on their influences on these systems. Several essential questions still remain unanswered: (1) Does a favorable or harmful effect of a given interleukin on diabetes necessarily imply similar effects on atherosclerosis? (2) Conversely, can the interleukins effects on atherosclerosis be extrapolated to diabetes? (3) Can the absence of interleukin activity on one of these diseases predict lack of effects on the other? We have addressed these questions, describing a novel interleukin classification based on their role in diabetes and cardiovascular disease [12].

Taking into account the alleged common inflammatory venue of these conditions, we hypothesize that the effects of each of the interleukins on both disorders will probably be moving in the same direction – regardless if harmful, favorable or neutral. If corroborated, this hypothesis could represent an additional step in building a unifying theory regarding the inflammatory basis of both type 2 diabetes and atherosclerosis.

How to Define, How to Classify

Interleukins are a wide spectrum of small regulatory protein molecules encompassed in the family of cytokines, exerting their effects via gene activation that leads to cellular stimulation, growth, differentiation, functional cell-surface receptor expression, and cellular effector function. In this regard, interleukins may exhibit marked effects on the regulation of immune responses and the pathogenesis of a great variety of diseases. Indeed, T cells have been categorized on the basis of the pattern of the interleukins that they secrete, resulting in either a cell-mediated immune response (TH1) or a humoral immune response (TH2) [13].

The interleukins are produced by a great variety of cells, mainly monocytes, macrophages, neutrophils, T cells, mast cells, and eosinophils. However, it must be pointed out that this is only a partial list. Endothelial and epithelial cells, fibroblasts, smooth muscle cells, neuronal cells, tumoral cells, etc., represent additional sources. Interleukins were cloned two decades ago and since then new members have been discovered in an ever-increasing number, the latest being the recently described IL-28 and IL-29 [14].

Attempts for grouping the interleukins according to predefined parameters may be done on the basis of the location of their activity. Thus, employing a site-based classification, interleukins are defined as:

(1) Autocrine: acting on the same cell that secretes the IL, like IL-10.
(2) Paracrine: acting on a cell located in an adjacent zone, like IL-12.
(3) Endocrine: secreted into the general circulation and acting far from its source, like IL-11.

This classification, while presenting some tutorial value, is imperfect because several interleukins overlap these categories.

Another possibility is to classify these compounds taking into account their biochemical influences. This generates a role-based classification, according to which interleukins will be:

(1) Proinflammatory: secreted mainly by mononuclear phagocytes in response to infectious agents, such as IL-1, IL-6 and IL-8.
(2) Immunoregulatory: involved in the activation, growth, and differentiation of lymphocytes and monocytes, like IL-2, IL-4 and IL-10.
(3) Leukocyte developmental: regulating immature white cell growth and differentiation; IL-3 and IL-7 represent this category.

This approach is also somewhat problematic, since it is more semantic than physiological. The term interleukin may be haphazard in some cases. For instance, IL-2 was formerly known as 'T cell growth factor' and IL-11 as 'adipogenesis inhibitory factor' [15]. On the other hand, several agents – like TNF-α1, the monocyte chemoattractant protein (MCP) isoforms and the transforming growth factor-β – whose functions are similar to those of interleukins, are not regarded as such. Thus, this nomenclature may be arbitrary.

From the standpoint of diabetes and cardiovascular medicine, the main concern with both the site-based and the role-based classifications is their lack of clinical significance. A practical approach would be to look at interleukins considering their influence on these systems – defined as benefit or damage – in the framework of an inflammatory process. This would be a yield-based classification, and in our opinion, preferable [12]. Like the former classifications, it allows definition of 3 categories:

(1) Noxious (the 'bad'): interleukins provoking a cascade of events ensuing in development of macrophages and foam cells, fatty streak formation and ultimately stable or unstable fibrous plaque. Proinflammatory stimuli such as oxidatively modified low density lipoprotein cholesterol, free radicals, cigarette smoking, elevated plasma homocysteine and infections, cause endothelial

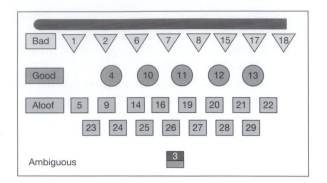

Fig. 1. Cardiovascular diabetologic approach to IL classification. The noxious ILs ('bad') are depicted as triangles, the protective ('good') as circles, and the aloof as squares. IL-3 is defined as ambiguous: albeit 'good' in terms of glucose metabolism, it was not clustered into this group due to its proarrhythmic effects on the heart. Modified from Fisman et al. [12].

dysfunction leading to compensatory responses which alter the normal properties of the endothelium. This cascade of events is mediated by proinflammatory and chemoattractant interleukins produced by activated inflammatory, vascular smooth muscle and endothelial cells. The fatty streak is the earliest manifestation of atherosclerosis, consisting mainly of monocyte-derived macrophages and T lymphocytes [16]. The noxious interleukins also show a consistent relation to diabetes via glucose regulation of monocyte adhesion [9] alongside etiopathogenic roles and increased genetic susceptibility to diabetic nephropathy [10, 17].

(2) Protective (the 'good'): interleukins representing a restraint for the development and progression of the atherothrombotic process. These compounds are involved in inhibition of proinflammatory agents production by activated monocytes or macrophages, suppression of IL-1, TNF-α and other cytokine activities, inhibition of matrix degrading MMP isoforms, reduction of tissue factor expression and inhibition of apoptosis of macrophages and monocytes after infection. In addition, in diabetic experimental models, administration of protective interleukins results in maintenance of euglycemia even in the absence of insulin [18].

(3) Aloof: this group includes interleukins whose influences on the cardiovascular system and on glucose metabolism are practically indifferent or not yet fully established.

The members of each of these groups are depicted in figure 1 and described in the following sections.

The 'Bad': Noxious Interleukins

This group comprises eight members: IL-1, IL-2, IL-6, IL-7, IL-8, IL-15, IL-17 and IL-18.

IL-1 is a glycoprotein which exists in two major biologically active isoforms, the predominantly membrane-bound IL-1α and the secreted IL-1β. Of these, IL-1β is the principally circulating isoform. Monocytes, macrophages and macrophage-derived foam cells are the main sources of IL-1, but it is also produced by others such as endothelial cells [19]. IL-1 mediates the inflammatory response occurring in the vascular wall during atherogenesis by activating monocytes and expression of adhesion molecules on endothelial cells, inducing secretion of other cytokines, chemokines and growth factors and stimulating smooth muscle cell proliferation [19]. It also induces coagulation [14]. As a key mediator of inflammation, IL-1 is plays a major role in the pathogenesis of CAD. Increased synthesis of IL-1 has been demonstrated in human arterial plaques [20], and serum concentrations of IL-1β are raised in patients with even minimal CAD [21]. In addition, IL-1β has deleterious effects on pancreatic islets and insulin-secreting β-cell lines. It is well established that it inhibits β-cell function and is cytotoxic to human and rodent pancreatic islets in vitro [22].

IL-2 is a T-cell-derived cytokine involved in the activation, growth, and differentiation of a variety of cells, including lymphocytes and monocytes. Attempting to determine the relationship between T lymphocyte activation and CAD by measuring plasma levels of cytokines related to T lymphocyte function in coronary patients, high levels of IL-2 and soluble IL-2 receptor were found in those with stable but not unstable angina [23]. It plays also a role in experimental diabetes. The nonobese diabetic mouse strain spontaneously develops autoimmune diabetes, which is characterized by insulitis, followed by selective destruction of β-cells in pancreatic islets. Evidence suggests that this β-cell destruction is mediated in part by IL-2; this cytokine was necessary and sufficient to direct naive T cells into the TH1 lineage [24].

IL-6 is a secondary multifunctional proinflammatory cytokine. It regulates humoral and cellular responses and plays a central role in inflammation and tissue injury. Its effects are mediated through interaction with its receptor complex, IL-6R. This cytokine plays a very important role in the pathogenesis of CAD. Large quantities of IL-6 are found in human atherosclerotic plaques [25]. IL-6 levels appear to be predictive of future CAD [26] and is elevated in patients with unstable angina compared with those with stable angina [27]. Patients with persistently elevated IL-6 levels demonstrate a worse in-hospital outcome following admission with unstable angina [28, 29]. IL-6 also plays a role in diabetes. It has been shown that postmenopausal women with type 1 diabetes present higher serum bioactive IL-6 levels than matched healthy controls [30]. Moreover, IL-6 polymorphism seems to be a genetic susceptibility factor for the progression of diabetic nephropathy [17]. In addition, we have recently shown that in patients with angina pectoris and/or healed myocardial infarction, a significantly higher risk for future cardiac events and mortality was found in the upper IL-6 quintile (odds ratio, 3.44; 95% CI 1.57–8.13) after a mean follow-up period of 6.3 years [31].

Recent data suggest a role for IL-7-driven inflammation in atherogenesis and the promotion of clinical instability in CAD involving interactions between platelets, monocytes, and chemokines [32]. This is based on the fact that its plasma levels were significantly increased in patients with stable, and – particularly – unstable angina compared to healthy controls; increased release from activated platelets appeared to be a major contributor to raised IL-7 levels in patients with angina. In addition, IL-7 enhanced the expression of several inflammatory chemokines in peripheral blood mononuclear cells in both healthy subjects and patients with CAD, and aspirin reduced both spontaneous and stimulated release of IL-7 from platelets [32]. Concerning diabetes, IL-7 is suggested to function through IL-2 production on mature T cells [15], which can lead to β-cell destruction.

IL-8 is a chemokine, or chemoattractant cytokine. Chemokines are members of a superfamily of small polypeptides mediating migration, growth and activation of leukocytes and a variety of other cells [33]. Chemokines are designated CC and CXC, according to the spacing of the first two of four conserved cysteine residues. MCP-1 is the prototype of the CC class, where the first two cysteines are adjacent, whereas IL-8 and the recently discovered fractalkine [34] are prototypes for the CXC class, in which the first two cysteines are separated by a single amino acid residue [33]. IL-8 is expressed by macrophages and released after inflammatory stimuli in response to the primary cytokines IL-1β and TNF-α. It induces chemoattraction of monocytes and activated T cells and can induce vascular smooth muscle cell proliferation and migration. In addition to causing local immune response, the recruited T cells along with macrophages occur in large numbers at the sites of plaque rupture, playing a major role in atherogenesis [35]. Inflammatory cytokines secreted by the T cells are capable of inducing the expression of several MMP isoforms by macrophages leading to development of unstable plaques. Moreover, IL-8 and the soluble form of selectin-P may be useful clinical predictors of unstable CAD [36]. Regarding glucose metabolism, monocyte MMP-1, MMP-3, and MMP-9 production are normal in type 2 diabetes [37], but plasma IL-8 concentrations after glucose load are increased in obese subjects with impaired fasting glucose in comparison to normoglycemic weight-matched individuals. These increased levels may be both insulin-mediated (by clamping) or glucose-mediated (during glucose tolerance test) [8]. Additionally, it is well established that glucose itself increases mono-cyte adhesion to human aortic endothelial cells [9].

IL-15 is a T cell growth factor that shares many functional similarities with IL-2, albeit no significant sequence homologies were found [15]; it has recently been shown to be present in tissue and organ allografts. IL-15 plays an impor-tant role in the rejection of a vascularized organ allograft and it was demon-strated that antagonists to IL-15 may be of therapeutic value in preventing allograft rejection [38]. In mice models, IL-15 is a cytokine leading to destruc-tive insulitis, as it elicits TH1-cytotoxic responses in both lymphoid and non-lymphoid immune cells and is unusually resistant to downregulation by antagonistic cytokines [39].

IL-17 is a T cell-derived cytokine that stimulates stromal cells and macrophages to secrete proinflammatory cytokines. It may harmfully influence diabetes and atherosclerosis due to its capability to induce the production of IL-6 and IL-8 [15]. In addition, it plays a role in alloimmune responses, shortening the survival of heterotopic heart transplantation in animals. Interference with this activity might suppress allograft rejection, representing a novel target for therapeutic intervention in heart transplant rejection [40]. In fact, IL-17 is a great family of isoforms sharing four highly conserved cysteine residues involved in the formation of intrachain disulfide linkages [41].

IL-18 – functionally related to IL-1 – is a proinflammatory cytokine with multiple biologic functions [42]. In concert with IL-12, IL-18 stimulates TH1-mediated immune responses. In addition, by itself it can stimulate TH2 cytokine production [42]. IL-18 plays a central role in orchestrating the cytokine cascade and accelerates atherosclerosis and plaque vulnerability in animal models. Serum IL-18 level was identified as a strong independent predictor of death from cardiovascular causes in patients with CAD regardless of the clinical status, strongly supporting recent experimental evidence of IL-18-mediated inflamma-tion leading to acceleration and vulnerability of atherosclerotic plaques [43]. Moreover, IL-18 is raised in heart failure patients, in whom elevations correlate with poorer cardiac functional class and higher TNF-α concentrations. IL-18 appears likely to participate in the pathophysiology of congestive heart failure [44]. Accumulating evidence suggests that this activity is supported by proin-flammatory cytokines such as TNF-α, IL-1β and IL-6. Cytokine actions directly identified to date include promotion of systemic catabolism, myocardial depres-sion, cardiac hypertrophy, and apoptosis of myocytes in congestive heart failure [44]. In the context of glucose metabolism, preclinical stages of type 1 diabetes are characterized by infiltrating T cells and by the peri- and intraislet accumula-tion of proinflammatory mediators [45]. Increased IL-18 expression is detected in islets during advanced stages of insulitis and correlates with elevated transcripts for interferon-γ and for the IL-18 receptor; the biological activity of

IL-18 is blocked using caspase inhibitors and anti-IL-18 antibodies. It is established that beta cells produce bioactive IL-18 in the course of insulitis and actively contribute to the exacerbation of inflammation leading to their own demise [45]. In addition, elevated levels of IL-18 and TNF-α in serum of patients with type 2 diabetes mellitus correlate with diabetic nephropathy [10].

The 'Good': Protective Interleukins

Five constituents are included in this category: IL-4, IL-10, IL-11, IL-12 and IL-13.

IL-4 is a cytokine of the T-helper 2 (TH2) subtype, mainly produced by activated T cells and mast cells. It is a pleiotropic cytokine that affects cells of multiple lineages, helping to stimulate antibody production. It possesses a striking ability to suppress proinflammatory responses such as IL-1 and TNF-α production [15]. In heart transplant recipients, relatively high frequencies of IL-4-producing T cells have a beneficial effect on the outcome, being associated with less rejection episodes [46]. This is manifested by IL-4 production within the donor heart, mainly by mast cells, and also by fibroblasts present in the donor's stromal elements [47]. Concerning diabetes, children with parents with type 1 diabetes demonstrated an impairment in the ability to produce the IL-4-related immunoglobulin G4 antibody response to tetanus toxoid [48]. This is consistent with a protective effect of IL-4 in early prediabetes [48]. In addition, the combined administration of IL-4/IL-10 expression plasmids has demonstrated synergistic effects on the prevention of autoimmune diabetes. On the cellular level, the chimeric IL-4 and IL-10 expression plasmid can effectively reduce the incidence of autoimmune insulitis [49].

IL-10 is secreted by activated monocytes/macrophages and lymphocytes, possessing multifaceted anti-inflammatory properties. Its secretion leads to suppressed cytokine production, to inhibition of MMP isoforms expression, and to blockage of apoptosis of macrophages and monocytes after infection. All these inflammatory mechanisms have been shown to play a pivotal role for atherosclerotic lesion development and progression, suggesting a beneficial regulatory role of IL-10. Indeed, numerous recent experimental studies have shown that either systemic or local IL-10 gene transfer not only attenuates atherogenesis, but also affects processes associated with lesion progression [50]. IL-10 is expressed in advanced human atherosclerosis and is associated with low inducible nitric oxide synthase expression and low levels of apoptosis, again suggesting a protective role of this anti-inflammatory cytokine [51]. A reduced IL-10 serum level is not only a marker of plaque instability favoring the development of acute coronary syndromes, but more importantly is indicative of a poor prognosis even after the occurrence of an acute ischemic event caused by plaque instability. In addition, the beneficial effect of elevated serum levels of IL-10 is restricted to patients with elevated CRP serum levels, indicative of an enhanced systemic inflammatory response [50]. With regard to diabetes, experimental studies using gene-targeted mice [52] provide direct evidence that IL-10 offers some protection against endothelial dysfunction during diabetes and that this effect is mediated by inhibition of increases in O_2^- in blood vessels. A source of this O_2^- may be xanthine oxidase. It was also demonstrated that endogenous IL-10 is an important counterbalance to mechanisms that produce endothelial dysfunction during diabetes [52] and that mucosal administration of IL-10 enhances oral tolerance in both autoimmune encephalomyelitis and diabetes [53]. These findings support the concept that IL-10 is also an important protective molecule in diabetes [51, 52].

Scarce data are available regarding the cardiac effects of IL-11. It was shown that myocytes and fibroblasts isolated from human atrium are able to secrete IL-6, IL-11 and leukemia inhibitory factor; IL-11 could be involved in autocrine and/or paracrine networks regulating myocardial cytoprotection [54]. The possibility of direct electrophysiologic effect on single human atrial myocytes was also considered, but not fully proved [55]. IL-11 presents interesting effects on diabetes, in which the inability of insulin to properly signal and stimulate the translocation of the insulin-responsive glucose transporter in muscle, adipocytes and liver leads to hyperglycemia. Adipose tissue has been identified as a site of synthesis and secretion of the proinflammatory cytokine TNF-α, which, acting in an autocrine manner, leads to insulin resistance. In this context, IL-11 emerges as an anti-inflammatory cytokine with receptors located on most cell types and tissues throughout the body, able to maintain euglycemia in the absence of insulin in animal models [9].

IL-12 is produced by various immune cells (e.g. monocytes, macrophages, dendritic cells, and neutrophils). It activates natural killer cells and cytotoxic T lymphocytes and induces the production of interferon-γ. IL-12 is associated with the cell-mediated immune response. It has been demonstrated to present protective effects in animal models of viral myocarditis [56]. This activity is enhanced by beta blockers, notably carvedilol, thus conferring a therapeutic benefit by upregulating the production of IL-12 and interferon-γ and by decreasing the virus load [56]. Moreover, IL-12 can significantly delay the rejection of allograft in a neonatal rat heart graft model, and this effect is mediated by nitric oxide production [57]. Initial data indicate a favorable action on glucose metabolism: lymphocyte T activation induced by IL-12 increases the expression of glucose transporter-like protein [58].

IL-13 is a cytokine primarily produced by the TH2 subset of lymphocytes that possesses powerful anti-inflammatory properties. It is synergistic with

IL-4, diminishes insulitis and is capable of downregulating immunoinflammatory diabetogenic pathways in nonobese diabetic mice, and further supports the concept that IL-4-related anti-inflammatory cytokines might play a role in the prevention of type 1 diabetes [59]. Regarding its cardiac aspects, proinflammatory cytokines participate in the worsening of cardiovascular function during heart failure, and their high circulating levels are related to the severity of myocardial dysfunction. Conversely, anti-inflammatory cytokines are believed to exhibit low values in these cases. In this context, plasma IL-13 was not detected at all in patients with heart failure [60].

The 'Aloof' Interleukins

This group of 15 includes the majority of interleukins known at present: IL-5, IL-9, IL-14, IL-16 and IL-19 through IL-29. Substantial effects on glucose metabolism and the cardiovascular system have not been described for these compounds.

IL-5, IL-9 and IL-16 are related to the respiratory system. IL-5 is mainly produced by activated T cells and appears to be required for the accumulation of eosinophils and airway hyperresponsiveness in the inflammatory lung [61]. IL-9 is known to regulate many cell types involved in TH2 responses classically associated with asthma, including B and T lymphocytes, mast cells, eosinophils and epithelial cells [62]. IL-16 is a lymphocyte chemoattractant factor bearing no structural resemblance to other cytokines or chemokines and its amino acid sequence is strongly preserved across species [63]. It is related to asthma and also able to inhibit human immunovirus replication [15].

IL-14 is a high-molecular-weight B cell growth factor. Autocrine or paracrine production of IL-14 may play a significant role in the rapid proliferation of non-Hodgkin's lymphoma [64].

IL-19, IL-20, IL-22 and IL-24 exhibit substantial sharing of receptor complexes. However, the biological effects of these four cytokines appear quite distinct: immune activity with IL-19, skin biology with IL-20, stimulation of production of acute-phase reactants with IL-22, and tumor apoptosis with IL-24 [65]. Despite the fact that they are structurally closely related to the 'good' IL-10, no protective effects have yet been described.

IL-21 induces the apoptosis of resting and activated primary B cells [66] and is a hepatocyte-stimulating factor [67]. Using gene-targeted mice lacking only IL-23, it was recently demonstrated that IL-23 is the critical cytokine for autoimmune inflammation of the brain [68]. IL-25 is derived from TH2 T cells. Infusion of mice with IL-25 induces IL-4, IL-5, and IL-13 gene expression, suggesting that IL-25 is capable of amplifying allergic type inflammatory responses by its actions on other cell types [69].

IL-26 is a T cell-derived cytokine, normally expressed at low levels but over-expressed after viral infection [14].

IL-27 is the newest addition to the 'good' IL-12 cytokine family, presenting specific stimulation on naive CD4+ T cells in both mice and humans and regulates the activity of B and T lymphocytes [70], but beneficial effects on diabetes or heart function were not yet described.

IL-28 and IL-29, distantly related to type I interferons, are induced by viral infection and show both antiviral and antimicrobial activity [14, 71].

Curtail of the Scope

It should be noted that the scope on interleukins depicted in this article presents several restrictions. These include genetic mapping, description of the numerous isoforms, characteristics of the interleukin receptors, general and specific antimicrobial and antiparasitic activities, role in tumoral and toxic diseases, etc. These issues were not discussed since they are beyond the span of this article. In addition, IL-3 was not included in any of the groups due to certain ambiguity. IL-3 – a hematopoietic and leukocyte developmental cytokine – shows multilineage colony-stimulating factor, augments alloreactive bone marrow-derived suppressor cell activity in vivo and in vitro, and is capable of regulating extrathymic T cell development from the bone marrow [15, 72]. It is a 'good' interleukin in terms of glucose metabolism, presenting defensive effects in experimental diabetes. Administration of IL-3 twice weekly starting at 2–4 weeks of age delayed the onset and reduced the overall incidence of diabetes in mice. Bone marrow cells obtained from IL-3-treated mice protected other mice from cyclophosphamide-induced diabetes [72]. On the other hand, in spontaneously contracting cultured cardiac myocytes, perfusion with IL-3 induced arrhythmias resulting in a complete cessation of spontaneous contractions and a severe loss of myocyte inotropy; the effects were concentration-dependent and reversible [73]. Thus, IL-3 appears to represent a special case, being the only interleukin whose effect is incongruous: protective for diabetes and noxious for the heart. However, it should be pointed out that such noxious effects do not include proinflammatory or atherogenic activities. IL-30 is in fact a protein that constitutes one of the chains of the heterodimeric IL-27. IL-31 presents a structure that places it in the family of cytokines being similar to IL-6, and may play a role in inflammation of the skin. IL-32 Induces monocytes and macrophages to secrete TNF-α and IL-8. IL-33 mediates its biological effects by interacting with the orphan IL-1 receptor, and activates the signaling pathways that drive production of IL-4, IL-5 and IL-13 [74]. IL-30 through 33 were not classified due to the scarce available data.

Matrixins

Matrixins, also named matrix metalloproteinases (MMPs), are prepro enzymes responsible for the timely breakdown of extracellular matrix (ECM). This is an essential process for embryonic development, morphogenesis, reproduction, and tissue resorption and remodeling. The expression of most matrixins is transcriptionally regulated by growth factors, hormones, cytokines, and cellular transformation. In addition, their proteolytic activity is precisely controlled during activation from their precursors and inhibition by endogenous inhibitors, α-macroglobulins, and tissue inhibitors of metalloproteinases (TIMPs) The TIMPs are specific inhibitors of matrixins that participate in controlling the local activities of MMPs in tissues [75]. This regulation is essential, since uncontrolled ECM remodeling of the myocardium and vasculature are features of cardiovascular disorders such as atherosclerosis, vascular stenosis, left ventricular hypertrophy, heart failure and aneurysms [76]. Various types of proteinases are implicated in ECM degradation, but the major enzymes are considered to be the matrixins. For the time being, 29 have been described in humans [77].

Biochemically, they belong to the family of zinc endopeptidases collectively referred to as metzincins. The metzincin superfamily is distinguished by a highly conserved motif containing three histidines that bind to zinc at the catalytic site and a conserved methionine that sits beneath the active site [78].

Classification

Based on domain organization and substrate preference, matrixins maybe grouped into five groups: collagenases, gelatinases, stromelysins, matrilysins, membrane-type (MT) matrixins. The are also several miscellaneous matrixins, not yet grouped in the above categories [79, 80].

Collagenases (like MMP-1, MMP-8, MMP-13 and MMP-18) are enzymes that are able to cleave the peptide bonds in the triple helical collagen molecule, and are characterized by specifically cleaving interstitial collagens I, II and III into 3/4 and 1/4 fragments, albeit they can digest other ECM molecules and soluble proteins. Recent studies indicated that MMP-1 activates protease-activated receptor (PAR)-1 by cleaving the same Arg-Ser bond cleaved by thrombins, which promotes growth and invasion of breast carcinoma cells [81]. Two other matrixins, i.e. MMP-2 and MMP-14 (MT1-MMP), also have collagenolytic activity, but they are classified into other subgroups because of their domain compositions. Collagenase has also been used in the isolation of cardiomyocytes suitable for the preparation of cultures. If tissue dissociation is accomplished by perfusion of the intact organ with enzyme solution, then collagenase is always the enzyme of choice, either alone or in combination with other enzymes such as hyaluronidase [82].

Gelatinases (as MMP-2 and MMP-9) readily digest gelatin with the help of their three fibronectin type II repeats that binds to gelatin/collagen. They also digest a number of ECM molecules including type IV, V and XI collagens, laminin, aggrecan core protein, etc. MMP-2, but not MMP-9, digests collagens I, II and III in a similar manner to the collagenases. The collagenolytic activity of MMP-2 is much weaker than MMP-1 in solution, but because proMMP-2 is recruited to the cell surface and activated. The association of a 92-kDa gelatinase with changes in left ventricular area suggests a possible modulating role for this matrix metalloproteinase in disruption of the fibrillar components of the left ventricular ECM [83].

Stromelysins (MMP-3, MMP-10 and MMP-11) have a domain arrangement similar to that of collagenases, but they do not cleave interstitial collagens. MMP-3 and MMP-10 are similar in structure and substrate specificity, but MMP- 11 (stromelysin 3) is distantly related. The MMP-11 gene is located on chromosome 22, whereas MMP-3 and MMP-10 are on chromosome 11, along with MMP-1, MMP-7, MMP-8, MMP-12, MMP-20, MMP-26 and MMP-27. MMP-3 and MMP-10 digest a number of ECM molecules and participate in pro-MMP activation. MMP-11, on the other hand, has very weak activity toward ECM molecules, but cleaves serpins more readily. MMP-11 has a furin recognition motif RX[R/K]R at the C-terminal end of the propeptide and therefore is activated intracellularly. An intracellular 40-kDa MMP-11 isoform (h-stromelysin 3) is found in cultured cells and placenta. This transcript, resulting from alternative splicing and promoter usage, lacks the signal peptide and the pro-domain. The function of this isoenzyme is not known. Its polymorphisms may not occur as independent events but rather be associated with other polymorphisms in the genome, such as cytokines and mediators of the inflammatory response, and may identify patients that are more vulnerable to adverse myocardial remodeling and, therefore, to a more rapid progression of the heart failure process [84].

Matrilysins (MMP-7 and MMP-26) are the smallest MMPs. They lack a hemopexin domain. MMP-7 is synthesized by epithelial cells and is secreted apically. Besides ECM components, MMP-7 processes cell-surface molecules such as pro-α-defensin, Fas-ligand, pro-TNF-α, and E-cadherin. MMP-26 is expressed in normal cells such as those of the endometrium and in some carcinomas. It digests several ECM molecules, and unlike most other MMPs, it is largely stored intracellularly. Surface plasmon resonance was used to document a direct MMP-7 interaction with connexin-43. Connexin-43 cleavage results in generation of a larger membrane-associated polypeptide and small free peptides derived from the extreme C-terminus of connexin-43. Thus, MM-7 affects connexin-43 levels, electrical conduction, and survival after myocardial infarction [85].

Membrane-type (MT) matrixins. There are six membrane-type MMPs (MT-MMPs): four are type I transmembrane proteins (MMP-14, MMP-15, MMP-16, and MMP-24), and two are glycosylphosphatidylinositol (GPI) anchored proteins (MMP-17 and MMP-25). With the exception of MT4-MMP, they are all capable of activating proMMP-2. These enzymes can also digest a number of ECM molecules, and MT1-MMP has collagenolytic activity on type I, II and·III collagens. MT1-MMP null mice exhibit skeletal abnormalities during postnatal development that are most likely due to lack of collagenolytic activity. MT1-MMP also plays an important role in angiogenesis. MT5-MMP is brain specific and is mainly expressed in the cerebellum. MT6-MMP (MMP-25) is expressed almost exclusively in peripheral blood leukocytes and in anaplastic astrocytomas and glioblastomas but not in meningiomas. MT matrixins are upregulated in kidneys of diabetic patients, suggesting a novel role for them in the pathogenesis of renal tubular atrophy and end-stage renal disease [86].

Implications

Atherosclerosis and diabetes present a pleiotropic progression in which inflammation appears to be a common background, and patients with diabetes experience accelerated atherosclerosis, which has been termed atheroscleropathy [87, 88]. Controlling the classical risk factors for CAD diminishes the incidence of both diseases. However, these risk factors are only partially successful in identifying many subjects who subsequently develop the ailments. The majority of myocardial infarctions are caused by coronary lesions presenting less than 50% luminal obstruction [89]. Moreover, lipid deposition in the endothelium, per se, does not explain the proliferation of smooth muscle cells during atherogenesis. These facts herald the concept that the plaque biology may be a very important determinant of disease outcome. In addition to the degree of vessel stenosis, biochemical processes within the plaque – such as those harvested by interleukins – are now widely recognized as a crucial aspect of stability. Moreover, sequelae of chronic hyperglycemia, such as oxidative stress and increased protein kinase C production, are widely invoked as pathogenic mechanisms for accelerated atherosclerosis [90].

Twenty-eight interleukins exhibit harmonized physiologic behavior regarding diabetes and atherosclerosis; each one presents converging effects on both diseases.

Eight interleukins are 'bad' (IL-1, IL-2, IL-6, IL-7, IL-8, IL-15, IL-17 and IL-18), five are 'good' (IL-4, IL-10, IL-11, IL-12 and IL-13), and the remaining fifteen are 'aloof'. According to this novel yield-based classification, the following implications may be drawn from the standpoint of cardiovascular diabetology: (1) a favorable effect of a given interleukin on either diabetes or atherosclerosis will predict a similar effect on the other; (2) equally, harmful interleukin effects on one disease can be extrapolated to the other, and (3) absence of influence of a given interleukin on one of these diseases forecasts lack of effects on the other.

Several studies report on substantial reductions in the incidence of type 2 diabetes during pharmacologic interventions aimed to treat CAD. Such results were observed with angiotensin-converting enzyme inhibitors [91, 92] and statins [93]. Reciprocally, antihyperglycemic agents like glitazones have shown favorable effects on nontraditional biomarkers of cardiovascular disease, suggesting the presence of antiatherogenic effects [94], and treating impaired glucose tolerance patients with acarbose was associated with a significant reduction in the risk of cardiovascular disease and hypertension [95]. Our present knowledge of the multifaceted physiological functions of interleukins allows the assumption that they play a pivotal role at the crossroad between glucose metabolism and atherothrombotic processes.

In principle, several matrixins with complementary substrate repertoires should be needed to mediate plaque rupture. Descriptive and correlative studies consistently demonstrate matrixins overexpression and matrix destruction at the macrophage-rich regions of atherosclerotic plaques that are prone to rupture. On the other hand, early fatty streaks also show upregulation of matrixins, which could therefore be involved in plaque building by intimal expansion as well as plaque rupture by matrix destruction. TIMPs are upregulated, especially at the base of plaques, and in part counteract the destructive potential of matrixins [76]. There has been a long-standing interest in the role of MMPs in cardiovascular disease. Numerous studies increased levels of MMPs at sites of atherosclerosis and aneurysm formation have been demonstrated [76].

The concept that the inflammatory process may play a leading role in the development of atherosclerotic plaques has led to the suggestion that secretion and activation of MMPs by macrophages induces degradation of ECM in the atherosclerotic plaque and plaque rupture. Based on these concepts, MMPs have been proposed to represent sensitive markers of inflammation in patients with coronary artery disease. The importance of collecting plasma rather than serum specimens for measuring MMPs in diagnostic testing has been stressed [96].

Similarly to interleukins, overepression of matrixins was documented in diabetes and its complications [97].

These facts further support the unifying etiologic theory of both ailments emphasizing the importance of a cardiovascular diabetologic approach to these cytokines for future research. Their targeting – in an attempt to develop pharmacologic activators of the 'good' interleukins, and inhibitors of the 'bad' ones – might provide an effective means to simultaneously control both atherosclerosis and diabetes mellitus.

References

1   Stern MP: Diabetes and cardiovascular disease: the 'common soil' hypothesis. Diabetes 1995;44: 369–374.
2   Tenenbaum A, Fisman EZ, Motro M: Metabolic syndrome and type 2 diabetes mellitus: focus on peroxisome proliferator activated receptors (PPAR). Cardiovasc Diabetol 2003;2:4.
3   Grundy SM, Benjamin IJ, Burke GL, Chait A, Eckel RH, Howard BV, Mitch W, Smith SC Jr, Sowers JR: Diabetes and cardiovascular disease: a statement for healthcare professionals from the American Heart Association. Circulation 1999;100:1134–1146.
4   Blake GJ, Ridker PM: Inflammatory bio-markers and cardiovascular risk prediction. J Intern Med 2002;252:283–294.
5   Alexander RW: Inflammation and coronary artery disease. N Engl J Med 1994;331:468–469.
6   Ross R: Atherosclerosis: an inflammatory disease. N Engl J Med 1999;340:115–126.
7   Libby P, Ridker PM, Maseri A: Inflammation and atherosclerosis. Circulation 2002;105: 1135–1143.
8   Straczkowski M, Kowalska I, Nikolajuk A, Dzienis-Straczkowska S, Szelachowska M, Kinalska I: Plasma interleukin 8 concentrations in obese subjects with impaired glucose tolerance. Cardiovasc Diabetol 2003;2:5.
9   Srinivasan S, Yeh M, Danziger EC, Hatley ME, Riggan AE, Leitinger N, Berliner JA, Hedrick CC: Glucose regulates monocyte adhesion through endothelial production of interleukin-8. Circ Res 2003;92:371–377.
10 Moriwaki Y, Yamamoto T, Shibutani Y, Aoki E, Tsutsumi Z, Takahashi S, Okamura H, Koga M, Fukuchi M, Hada T: Elevated levels of interleukin-18 and tumor necrosis factor-alpha in serum of patients with type 2 diabetes mellitus: relationship with diabetic nephropathy. Metabolism 2003;52:605–608.
11 Pradhan AD, Ridker PM: Do atherosclerosis and diabetes share a common inflammatory basis? Eur Heart J 2002;23:831–834.
12 Fisman EZ, Motro M, Tenenbaum A: Cardiovascular diabetology in the core of a novel interleukins classification: the bad, the good and the aloof. Cardiovasc Diabetol 2003;2:11.
13 Herman A, Kappler JW, Marrack P, Pullen AM: Superantigens: mechanism of T-cell stimulation and role in immune responses. Annu Rev Immunol 1991;9:745–772.
14 Gadina M, Ferguson PR, Johnston JA: New interleukins: are there any more? Curr Opin Infect Dis 2003;16:211–217.
15 Curfs JH, Meis JF, Hoogkamp-Korstanje JA: A primer on cytokines: sources, receptors, effects, and inducers. Clin Microbiol Rev 1997;10:742–780.
16 Stary HC, Chandler AB, Glagov S, Guyton JR, Insull W Jr, Rosenfeld ME, Schaffer SA, Schwartz CJ, Wagner WD, Wissler RW: A definition of initial, fatty streak, and intermediate lesions of atherosclerosis: a report from the Committee on Vascular Lesions of the Council on Arteriosclerosis, American Heart Association. Circulation 1994;89:2462–2478.
17 Kitamura A, Hasegawa G, Obayashi H, Kamiuchi K, Ishii M, Yano M, Tanaka T, Yamaguchi M, Shigeta H, Ogata M, Nakamura N, Yoshikawa T: Interleukin-6 polymorphism (−634C/G) in the promotor region and the progression of diabetic nephropathy in type 2 diabetes. Diabet Med 2002;19:1000–1005.
18 Tenney R, Turnbull JR, Stansfield KA, Pekala PH: The regulation of adipocyte metabolism and gene expression by interleukin-11. Adv Enzyme Regul 2003;43:153–166.
19 Dinarello CA, Wolff SM: The role of interleukin-1 in disease. N Engl J Med 1993;328:106–113.

20 Tipping PG, Hancock WW: Production of tumor necrosis factor and interleukin-1 by macrophages from human atheromatous plaques. Am J Pathol 1991;138:951–960.

21 Hasdai D, Scheinowitz M, Leibovitz E, Sclarovsky S, Eldar M, Barak V: Increased serum concentrations of interleukin-1 beta in patients with coronary artery disease. Heart 1996;76:24–28.

22 Major CD, Wolf BA: Interleukin-1beta stimulation of c-Jun NH(2)-terminal kinase activity in insulin-secreting cells: evidence for cytoplasmic restriction. Diabetes 2001;50:2721–2728.

23 Simon AD, Yazdani S, Wang W, Schwartz A, Rabbani LE: Elevated plasma levels of interleukin-2 and soluble IL-2 receptor in ischemic heart disease. Clin Cardiol 2001;24:253–256.

24 Zhou W, Zhang F, Aune TM: Either IL-2 or IL-12 is sufficient to direct Th1 differentiation by nonobese diabetic T cells. J Immunol 2003;170:735–740.

25 Rus HG, Vlaicu R, Niculescu F: Interleukin-6 and interleukin-8 protein and gene expression in human arterial atherosclerotic wall. Atherosclerosis 1996;127:263–271.

26 Harris TB, Ferrucci L, Tracy RP, Corti MC, Wacholder S, Ettinger WH Jr, Heimovitz H, Cohen HJ, Wallace R: Mortality risk associated with elevated interleukin-6 and C-reactive protein in old age. Am J Med 1999;196:506–512.

27 Biasucci LM, Vitelli A, Liuzzo G, Altamura S, Caligiuri G, Monaco C, Rebuzzi AG, Ciliberto G, Maseri A: Elevated levels of IL-6 in unstable angina. Circulation 1996;94:874–877.

28 Biasucci LM, Liuzzo G, Grillo RL, Caligiuri G, Rebuzzi AG, Buffon A, Summaria F, Ginnetti F, Fadda G, Maseri A: Elevated levels of C-reactive protein at discharge predicts recurrent instability in patients with unstable angina. Circulation 1999;99:855–860.

29 Biasucci LM, Liuzzo G, Fantuzzi G, Caligiuri G, Rebuzzi AG, Ginnetti F, Dinarello CA, Maseri A: Increasing levels of interleukin (IL)-1Ra and IL-6 during the first 2 days of hospitalization in unstable angina are associated with increased risk of in-hospital coronary events. Circulation 1999;88:2079–2084.

30 Rachon D, Mysliwska J, Suchecka-Rachon K, Semetkowska-Jurkiewicz B, Zorena K, Lysiak-Szydlowska W: Serum interleukin-6 levels and bone mineral density at the femoral neck in post-menopausal women with type 1 diabetes. Diabet Med 2003;20:475–480.

31 Fisman EZ, Benderly M, Esper RJ, Behar S, Boyko V, Adler Y, Tanne D, Matas Z, Tenenbaum A: Interleukin-6 and the risk of future cardiovascular events in patients with angina pectoris and/or healed myocardial infarction. Am J Cardiol 2006;98:14–18.

32 Damas JK, Waehre T, Yndestad A, Otterdal K, Hognestad A, Solum NO, Gullestad L, Froland SS, Aukrust P: Interleukin-7-mediated inflammation in unstable angina: possible role of chemokines and platelets. Circulation 2003;107:2670–2676.

33 Saadeddin SM, Habbab MA, Ferns GA: Markers of inflammation and coronary artery disease. Med Sci Monit 2002;8:RA5–RA12.

34 Wong BW, Wong D, McManus BM: Characterization of fractalkine (CX3CL1) and CX3CR1 in human coronary arteries with native atherosclerosis, diabetes mellitus, and transplant vascular disease. Cardiovasc Pathol 2002;11:332–338.

35 Gerszten RE, Garcia-Zepeda EA, Lim YC, Yoshida M, Ding HA, Gimbrone MA Jr, Luster AD, Luscinskas FW, Rosenzweig A: MCP-1 and IL-8 trigger firm adhesion of monocytes to vascular endothelium under flow conditions. Nature 1999;398:718–723.

36 Romuk E, Skrzep-Poloczek B, Wojciechowska C, Tomasik A, Birkner E, Wodniecki J, Gabrylewicz B, Ochala A, Tendera M: Selectin-P and interleukin-8 plasma levels in coronary heart disease patients. Eur J Clin Invest 2002;32:657–661.

37 Baugh MD, Gavrilovic J, Davies IR, Hughes DA, Sampson MJ: Monocyte matrix metalloproteinase production in type 2 diabetes and controls: a cross-sectional study. Cardiovasc Diabetol 2003;2:3.

38 Smith XG, Bolton EM, Ruchatz H, Wei X, Liew FY, Bradley JA: Selective blockade of IL-15 by soluble IL-15 receptor alpha-chain enhances cardiac allograft survival. J Immunol 2000;165:3444–3450.

39 Rothe H, Hausmann A, Kolb H: Immunoregulation during disease progression in prediabetic NOD mice: inverse expression of arginase and prostaglandin H synthase 2 vs. interleukin-15. Horm Metab Res 2002;34:7–12.

40 Antonysamy MA, Fanslow WC, Fu F, Li W, Qian S, Troutt AB, Thomson AW: Evidence for a role of IL-17 in organ allograft rejection: IL-17 promotes the functional differentiation of dendritic cell progenitors. J Immunol 1999;162:577–584.

41 Starnes T, Broxmeyer HE, Robertson MJ, Hromas R: Cutting edge: IL-17D, a novel member of the IL-17 family, stimulates cytokine production and inhibits hemopoiesis. J Immunol 2002;169: 642–646.

42 Nakanishi K, Yoshimoto T, Tsutsui H, Okamura H: Interleukin-18 regulates both Th1 and Th2 responses. Annu Rev Immunol 2001;19:423–474.

43 Blankenberg S, Tiret L, Bickel C, Peetz D, Cambien F, Meyer J, Rupprecht HJ, AtheroGene Investigators: Interleukin-18 is a strong predictor of cardiovascular death in stable and unstable angina. Circulation 2002;106:24–30.

44 Naito Y, Tsujino T, Fujioka Y, Ohyanagi M, Okamura H, Iwasaki T: Increased circulating interleukin-18 in patients with congestive heart failure. Heart 2002;88:296–297.

45 Frigerio S, Hollander GA, Zumsteg U: Functional IL-18 is produced by primary pancreatic mouse islets and NIT-1 beta cells and participates in the progression towards destructive insulitis. Horm Res 2002;57:94–104.

46 Bijlsma FJ, vanKuik J, Marcel BS, Tilanus GJ, deJonge N, Rozemuller EH, van den Tweel JG, Gmelig-Meyling FHJ, deWeger RA: Donor interleukin-4 promoter gene polymorphism influences allograft rejection after heart transplantation. J Heart Lung Transplant 2002;21:340–346.

47 van Hoffen E, Polen E, Robertus-Teunissen M, De Jonge N, Lahpor JR, Gmelig-Meyling FH, De Weger RA: High frequency of IL-4 producing helper T lymphocytes associated with a reduced incidence of heart allograft rejection. Transpl Int 2000;13(suppl 1):216–224.

48 Schmid S, Molteni A, Fuchtenbusch M, Naserke HE, Ziegler AG, Bonifacio E: Reduced IL-4 associated antibody responses to vaccine in early pre-diabetes. Diabetologia 2002;45:677–685.

49 Lee M, Ko KS, Oh S, Kim SW: Prevention of autoimmune insulitis by delivery of a chimeric plasmid encoding interleukin-4 and interleukin-10. J Control Release 2003;88:333–342.

50 Heeschen C, Dimmeler S, Hamm CW, Fichtlscherer S, Boersma E, Simoons ML, Zeiher AM, for the CAPTURE Study Investigators: Serum level of the anti-inflammatory cytokine interleukin-10 is an important prognostic determinant in patients with acute coronary syndromes. Circulation 2003;107:2109–2114.

51 Mallat Z, Heymes C, Ohan J, Faggin E, Leseche G, Tedgui A: Expression of interleukin-10 in advanced human atherosclerotic plaques: relation to inducible nitric oxide synthase expression and cell death. Arterioscler Thromb Vasc Biol 1999;19:611–616.

52 Gunnett CA, Heistad DD, Faraci FM: Interleukin-10 protects nitric oxide-dependent relaxation during diabetes: role of superoxide. Diabetes 2002;51:1931–1937.

53 Slavin AJ, Maron R, Weiner HL: Mucosal administration of IL-10 enhances oral tolerance in autoimmune encephalomyelitis and diabetes. Int Immunol 2001;13:825–833.

54 Ancey C, Corbi P, Froger J, Delwail A, Wijdenes J, Gascan H, Potreau D, Lecron JC: Secretion of IL-6, IL-11 and LIF by human cardiomyocytes in primary culture. Cytokine 2002;18: 199–205.

55 Sartiani L, De Paoli P, Lonardo G, Pino R, Conti AA, Cerbai E, Pelleg A, Belardinelli L, Mugelli A: Does recombinant human interleukin-11 exert direct electrophysiologic effects on single human atrial myocytes? J Cardiovasc Pharmacol 2002;39:425–434.

56 Nishio R, Shioi T, Sasayama S, Matsumori A: Carvedilol increases the production of interleukin-12 and interferon-gamma and improves the survival of mice infected with the encephalomyocarditis virus. J Am Coll Cardiol 2003;41:340–345.

57 Verma N, He XY, Chen J, Robinson C, Boyd R, Tran G, Hall BM: Interleukin 12 delays allograft rejection: effect mediated via nitric oxide. Transplant Proc 2001;33:416–417.

58 Li B, Cao D, Xu H, Chang J, Zhou G, Tian J, Li D, Theze J, Wu C: Interleukin-12 induces gene expression in interleukin-2 stimulated human T lymphocytes. Eur Cytokine Netw 2000;11: 602–607.

59 Zaccone P, Phillips J, Conget I, Gomis R, Haskins K, Minty A, Bendtzen K, Cooke A, Nicoletti F: Interleukin-13 prevents autoimmune diabetes in NOD mice. Diabetes 1999;48:1522–1528.

60 Masson S, Latini R, Bevilacqua M, Vago T, Sessa F, Torri M, Anesini A, Salio M, Pasotti E, Agnello D, et al: Within-patient variability of hormone and cytokine concentrations in heart failure. Pharmacol Res 1998;37:213–217.

61 Matsumoto N, Katoh S, Mukae H, Matsuo T, Takatsu K, Matsukura S: Critical role of IL-5 in antigen-induced pulmonary eosinophilia, but not in lymphocyte activation. Int Arch Allergy Immunol 2003;130:209–215.

62   Pilette C, Ouadrhiri Y, Van Snick J, Renauld JC, Staquet P, Vaerman JP, Sibille Y: Oxidative burst in lipopolysaccharide-activated human alveolar macrophages is inhibited by interleukin-9. Eur Respir J 2002;20:1198–1205.

63   Parada NA, Cruikshank WW, Danis HL, Ryan TC, Center DM: IL-16 and other CD4 ligand-induced migration is dependent upon protein kinase C. Cell Immunol 1996;168:100–106.

64   Ford R, Tamayo A, Martin B, Niu K, Claypool K, Cabanillas F, Ambrus J Jr: Identification of B-cell growth factors (interleukin-14; high molecular weight B-cell growth factors) in effusion fluids from patients with aggressive B-cell lymphomas. Blood 1995;86:283–293.

65   Parrish-Novak J, Xu W, Brender T, Yao L, Jones C, West J, Brandt C, Jelinek L, Madden K, McKernan PA, et al: Interleukins 19, 20, and 24 signal through two distinct receptor complexes: differences in receptor-ligand interactions mediate unique biological functions. J Biol Chem 2002;277:47517–47523.

66   Mehta DS, Wurster AL, Whitters MJ, Young DA, Collins M, Grusby MJ: IL-21 induces the apoptosis of resting and activated primary B cells. J Immunol 2003;170:4111–4118.

67   Dumoutier L, Van Roost E, Colau D, Renauld JC: Human interleukin-10-related T cell-derived inducible factor: molecular cloning and functional characterization as an hepatocyte-stimulating factor. Proc Natl Acad Sci USA 2000;97:10144–10149.

68   Cua DJ, Sherlock J, Chen Y, Murphy CA, Joyce B, Seymour B, Lucian L, To W, Kwan S, Churakova T, et al: Interleukin-23 rather than interleukin-12 is the critical cytokine for autoimmune inflammation of the brain. Nature 2003;421:744–748.

69   Fort MM, Cheung J, Yen D, Li J, Zurawski SM, Lo S, Menon S, Clifford T, Hunte B, Lesley R, et al: IL-25 induces IL-4, IL-5, and IL-13 and Th2-associated pathologies in vivo. Immunity 2001;15:985–995.

70   Cordoba-Rodriguez R, Frucht DM: IL-23 and IL-27: new members of the growing family of IL-12-related cytokines with important implications for therapeutics. Expert Opin Biol Ther 2003;3:715–723.

71   Sheppard P, Kindsvogel W, Xu W, Henderson K, Schlutsmeyer S, Whitmore TE, Kuestner R, Garrigues U, Birks C, Roraback J, et al: IL-28, IL-29 and their class II cytokine receptor IL-28R. Nat Immunol 2003;4:63–68.

72   Ito A, Aoyanagi N, Maki T: Regulation of autoimmune diabetes by interleukin 3-dependent bone marrow-derived cells in NOD mice. J Autoimmun 1997;10:331–338.

73   Weisensee D, Bereiter-Hahn J, Schoeppe W, Low-Friedrich I: Effects of cytokines on the contractility of cultured cardiac myocytes. Int J Immunopharmacol 1993;15:581–587.

74   Schmitz J, Owyang A, Oldham E, Song Y, Murphy E, McClanahan TK, Zurawski G, Moshrefi M, Qin J, Li X, Gorman DM, Bazan JF, Kastelein RA: IL-33, an interleukin-1-like cytokine that signals via the IL-1 receptor-related protein ST2 and induces T helper type 2-associated cytokines. Immunity 2005;23:479–490.

75   Nagase H, Woessner JF: Matrix metalloproteinases. J Biol Chem 1999;274:21491–21494.

76   Newby AC: Dual role of matrix metalloproteinases (matrixins) in intimal thickening and atherosclerotic plaque rupture. Physiol Rev 2005;85:1–31.

77   Verma RP, Hansch C: Matrix metalloproteinases (MMPs): chemical-biological functions and (Q)SARs. Bioorg Med Chem 2007;15:2223–2268.

78   Stoker W, Bode W: Structural features of a superfamily of zinc-endopeptidases: the metzincins. Curr Opin Str Biol 1995;5:383–390.

79   Visse R, Nagase H: Matrix metalloproteinases and tissue inhibitors of metalloproteinases: structure, function, and biochemistry. Circ Res 2003;92:827–839.

80   Nagase H, Visse R, Murphy G: Structure and function of matrix metalloproteinases and TIMPs. Cardiovasc Res 2006;69:562–573.

81   Boire A, Covic L, Agarwal A, Jacques S, Sherifi S, Kuliopulos A: PAR1 is a matrix metalloprotease-1 receptor that promotes invasion and tumorigenesis of breast cancer cells. Cell 2005;120:303–313.

82   Nag AC, Cheng M: Adult mammalian cardiac muscle cells in culture. Tissue Cell 1981;13:515–523.

83   Armstrong PW, Moe GW, Howard RJ, Grima EA, Cruz TF: Structural remodelling in heart failure: gelatinase induction. Can J Cardiol 1994;10:214–220.

84   Spinale FG: Matrix metalloproteinase gene polymorphisms in heart failure: new pieces to the myocardial matrix puzzle. Eur Heart J 2004;25:631–633.

85 Lindsey ML, Escobar GP, Mukherjee R, Goshorn DK, Sheats NJ, Bruce JA, Mains IM, Hendrick JK, Hewett KW, Gourdie RG, Matrisian LM, Spinale FG: Matrix metalloproteinase-7 affects connexin-43 levels, electrical conduction, and survival after myocardial infarction. Circulation 2006;113:2919–2928.

86 Romanic AM, Burns-Kurtis CL, Ao Z, Arleth AJ, Ohlstein EH: Upregulated expression of human membrane type-5 matrix metalloproteinase in kidneys from diabetic patients. Am J Physiol 2001;281:F309–F317.

87 Hayden MR, Tyagi SC: Intimal redox stress: accelerated atherosclerosis in metabolic syndrome and type 2 diabetes mellitus. Atheroscleropathy Cardiovasc Diabetol 2002;1:3.

88 Hayden MR, Tyagi SC: Is type 2 diabetes mellitus a vascular disease (atheroscleropathy) with hyperglycemia a late manifestation? The role of NOS, NO, and redox stress. Cardiovasc Diabetol 2003;2:2.

89 Fuster V: Mechanisms leading to myocardial infarction: insights from studies of vascular biology. Circulation 1994;90:2126–2146.

90 Aronson D, Rayfield EJ: How hyperglycemia promotes atherosclerosis: molecular mechanisms. Cardiovasc Diabetol 2002;1:1.

91 Hansson L, Lindholm LH, Niskanen L, Lanke J, Hedner T, Niklason A, Luomanmaki K, Dahlof B, de Faire U, Morlin C, et al: Effect of angiotensin-converting-enzyme inhibition compared with conventional therapy on cardiovascular morbidity and mortality in hypertension: the Captopril Prevention Project (CAPPP) randomised trial. Lancet 1999;353:611–616.

92 Yusuf S, Sleight P, Pogue J, Bosch J, Davies R, Dagenais G: Effects of an angiotensin-converting-enzyme inhibitor, ramipril, on cardiovascular events in high-risk patients. The Heart Outcomes Prevention Evaluation Study Investigators. N Engl J Med 2000;342:145–153.

93 Freeman DJ, Norrie J, Sattar N, Neely RD, Cobbe SM, Ford I, Isles C, Lorimer AR, Macfarlane PW, McKillop JH, et al: Pravastatin and the development of diabetes mellitus: evidence for a protective treatment effect in the West of Scotland Coronary Prevention Study. Circulation 2001;103: 357–362.

94 Haffner SM, Greenberg AS, Weston WM, Chen H, Williams K, Freed MI: Effect of rosiglitazone treatment on nontraditional markers of cardiovascular disease in patients with type 2 diabetes mellitus. Circulation 2002;106:679–684.

95 Chiasson JL, Josse RG, Gomis R, Hanefeld M, Karasik A, Laakso M, STOP-NIDDM Trial Research Group: Acarbose treatment and the risk of cardiovascular disease and hypertension in patients with impaired glucose tolerance: the STOP-NIDDM trial. JAMA 2003;290:486–494.

96 van den Steen PE, Dubois B, Nelissen I, Rudd PM, Dwek RA, Opdenakker G: Biochemistry and molecular biology of gelatinase B or matrix metalloproteinase-9 (MMP-9). Crit Rev Biochem Mol Biol 2002;37:376–536.

97 Marx N, Froehlich J, Siam L, Ittner J, Wierse G, Schmidt A, Scharnagl H, Hombach V, Koenig W: Antidiabetic PPAR gamma-activator rosiglitazone reduces MMP-9 serum levels in type 2 diabetic patients with coronary artery disease. Arterioscler Thromb Vasc Biol 2003;23:283–288.

Prof. Enrique Z. Fisman
Cardiovascular Diabetology Research Foundation
Holon 58484 (Israel)
E-Mail zfisman@post.tau.ac.il

Fisman EZ, Tenenbaum A (eds): Cardiovascular Diabetology: Clinical, Metabolic and Inflammatory Facets. Adv Cardiol. Basel, Karger, 2008, vol 45, pp 65–81

....

Arterial Elasticity in Cardiovascular Disease: Focus on Hypertension, Metabolic Syndrome and Diabetes

Relu Cernes[a,d]   *Reuven Zimlichman*[b,d]   *Marina Shargorodsky*[c,d]

Departments of [a]Nephrology, [b]Medicine, [c]Endocrinology and Diabetes, and [d]The Brunner Institute for Cardiovascular Research, Wolfson Medical Center, Holon, and Sackler School of Medicine, Tel-Aviv University, Tel-Aviv, Israel

Abstract

Arterial stiffness is an independent risk factor for premature cardiovascular morbidity and mortality that can be evaluated by noninvasive methods and can be reduced by good clinical management. The present chapter examines the association between arterial stiffness and cardiovascular risk factors including hypertension, metabolic syndrome, diabetes, advanced renal failure, hypercholesterolemia and obesity. The mechanisms responsible for the structural and functional modifications of the arterial wall are also described. We deal with parameters related to arterial compliance, focusing on two of them, pulse wave velocity and the augmentation index, useful in rapid assessment of arterial compliance by the bedside. Data that highlight the role of aortic pulse wave velocity and the augmentation index as independent factors in predicting fatal and nonfatal cardiovascular events in different populations are briefly presented. A number of lifestyle changes and traditional antihypertensive agents that improve arterial compliance are finally discussed. Novel therapies, such as statins, thiazolidindinediones, phosphodiesterase inhibitors and inhibitors or breakers of advanced glycation end product cross-links between colagen and elastin hold substantial promise.

The principal function of the arterial system is to deliver an adequate supply of blood to the tissues and organs. In performing this conduit function, the arteries transform the pulsatile flow generated by ventricular contraction into a continuous flow of blood in the periphery. This latter cushioning function is dependent on the mechanical properties of the arterial wall. Arterial compliance depends on the structure and function of the vessel wall.

Arterial Wall and Arterial Compliance

Arterial Wall

The arterial wall is formed by endothelium, intima, media and adventitia. The endothelial basement membrane (BM) is the main support for attachment of endothelial cells and provides a filtering mechanism due to strong anionic charges of its matrix. The extracellular matrix (ECM) consists of collagen, elastin, proteoglycans (glycosaminoglycans), hyaluronan and structural adhesive glycoproteins. All these components are under the control of metalloproteinases.

The endothelial cells and BM along with ECM are the first defense mechanism against various toxic stimuli: aldosterone, LDL cholesterol, viruses and so on.

Therefore, ECM is the first layer that is affected by the process of atherogenesis. Later, each layer will be affected by these injurious stimuli. We will briefly describe the ECM components.

Collagen

Collagen is the most abundant protein. The collagen molecule is formed by three polypeptide chains, which intertwine to form triple-helical rope-like collagen fibrils. These fibrils are cross-linked by hydroxyl groups between alpha chains (a major contributor to their tensile strength) to form the collagen fiber. These fibers, in turn, form collagen bundles. Gaps in the collagen fibril give the cross-banding appearance of type I and II collagen fibers at a characteristic length of 67 nm when viewed by electron microscopy. In type III collagen there is a structurally beaded appearance instead of the characteristic cross-banding appearance observed in type I and II collagen. The physical and tensile strength of collagens is typified by collagen type I (having the tensile strength of steel), which predominates in bones, tendons, skin, and mature scars, while type II collagen is thinner and predominates in cartilage, vitreous humor and nucleus pulposus. Type III collagen is found in organs requiring more plasticity such as blood vessels, heart, gastrointestinal tract, uterus, and the dermis. Types I, II and III collagen are the fibrillar-interstitial collagens and are the most abundant collagen types. They are important in diabetic remodeling fibrosis within the myocardium, the tubulointerstitium of the kidney, the intima in atheroscleropathy, dermopathy, interstitial changes within the retina (retinopathy), and possibly the neuronal unit of neuropathy. In contrast, collagens IV, V, and VI are nonfibrillar or amorphous and are found in BMs and interstitial tissue.

One very unique feature of type IV collagen is the presence of 7–8 cysteine residues, which are involved in intra- and intermolecular disulfide bonds, which aid in the stabilization of this polymer. This presence of cysteine in type

IV collagen is in contrast to mature fibrillar collagens types I, II and III, as they lack a cysteine moiety. Type IV collagen is found exclusively in BM [1–3].

Elastin

Elastin is known to provide support and elasticity. This elasticity is important for many tissues and organs such as the blood vessels, heart, skin, lung, and uterus. Elastin is a 70-kDa glycoprotein and constitutes the central core of elastic fibers. It is cross-linked, but unlike most other proteins it does not form definite folds but rather oscillates between different states to form random coils. It is this cross-linked, random-coiled structure of elastin that determines the capacity of the elastic network to stretch and rebound.

Elastin provides an elastic molecular rebound capacity to the ECM and this is why there is a distinct internal and external elastic lamina on either side of the medial vascular smooth muscle layer of the arterial vessel wall [1–3].

Proteoglycan

Proteoglycan (PG) is found within the intima. It is synthesized primarily by the vascular smooth muscle cell and in BM by the endothelium. PG consist of core protein(s) covalently linked to one or more highly sulfated polysaccharide chains, called glycosaminoglycans. These molecules are highly diverse with multiple combinations of core proteins and polysaccharide chains. Examples are: heparan sulfate proteoglycans, chondroitin sulfate proteoglycans, keratan sulfate proteoglycans, and dermatan sulfate proteoglycans [1–3].

Hyaluronan

Hyaluronan is a huge molecule formed by disaccharides stretched end-to-end, while lacking a core protein. It binds large amounts of water and forms a viscous hydrated gel, which gives the ECM turgor and allows it to resist compressive forces. Because of this unique ability it is found in abundance in cartilage of joints as it provides resilience and lubrication. It serves as a ligand for core proteins and is often a backbone for large proteoglycan complexes. It facilitates cell migration and inhibits cell-cell adhesion. Hyaluronan is increased in atherosclerotic plaque erosion and is decreased in the vulnerable thin-cap atheroma associated with plaque rupture [1–3].

Structural-Adhesive Glycoproteins

Fibronectin forms a primitive matrix that allows the initial organization to be replaced by the definitive, organ-specific matrix. Fibronectin is a multifunctional adhesive protein whose primary function is to attach cells to a variety of matrices. Structurally, it consists of two polypeptide chains held together by two disulfide bonds. In addition to providing structural support it is associated with cell surfaces and BMs.

Laminin is the most abundant glycoprotein in BMs. This structural-adhesive glycoprotein binds to cells, proteoglycans, and type IV collagen. Laminin is a hetero-trimeric polypeptide and appears as a cross-like structure with a single central polypeptide A chain and two flanking polypeptide B chains. This adhesive glycoprotein is felt to be important in cellular alignment [1–3].

Metalloproteinases and Their Inhibitors

Collagen is maintained under the control of a group of zinc dependent, redox sensitive endopeptidases, named metalloproteinases. There is a delicate balance between the tearing down, rebuilding, tailoring and remodeling of the collagens within ECM. Also there is a delicate balance between metallopro-teinases and their inhibitors. In physiological conditions, homeostasis is achieved. But, when the balance is broken, metalloproteinases degrade collagen and hydrolyze elastin, which results in rupture of arterial wall vulnerable plaques [1–3].

Systolic Hypertension, Wide Pulse Pressure, Central Artery Stiffness and Arterial Compliance

Systolic hypertension results principally from increased aortic and central arterial stiffness, although peripheral vasoconstriction also contributes [4].

The clinical hallmark of systolic hypertension is a pattern of wide pulse pressure (PP). PP is defined as the difference between systolic blood pressure (SBP) and diastolic blood pressure (DBP). In young healthy people the elastic recoil of proximal aorta and large arteries dampens the impact of pulsatile flow (narrow PP) by retaining a fraction of each cardiac stroke volume during systole and then delivering this retained volume in diastole.

When central arteries stiffen with age and hypertension, the full stroke volume is delivered through the resistance arterioles during systole because there is no elastic recoil (compliance) of the aorta. As a result, the PP widens and the SBP rises, independent of cardiac output or systemic resistance [4–7].

The arterial stiffness is altered primarily in association with increased collagen content and alterations of extracellular matrix and calcification of the arterial wall [9]. Arterial stiffness is one of the principal factors opposing left ventricular ejection. Arterial stiffening increases left ventricular afterload and alters the coronary perfusion and is a strong independent factor associated with morbidity and mortality, in the general population as well as in people suffering from cardiovascular disease and chronic renal failure [4–7].

Compliance defines the capacitive properties of central arteries, whose role it is to dampen pressure and flow oscillations and to transform pulsatile flow and pressure in arteries into a steady flow and pressure in peripheral tissues. Stiffness is the reciprocal value of compliance [4–8].

Assessment of Arterial Stiffness: Measurement of Pulse-Wave Velocity and Augmentation Index

Several parameters of arterial stiffness have been investigated. The shift in importance from diastolic to systolic hypertension has prompted the development of new methods to evaluate arterial compliance. Two of these, derived from the application of applanation tonometry, have emerged as particularly valuable: pulse-wave velocity (PWV) and the augmentation index (AI). Their merits are a simple method of calculation/measurement, reproducible values, and prospectively validated prognostic significance.

PWV is greater in stiffer arteries, and is clearly associated with increased mortality in populations with cardiovascular disease or chronic kidney disease. PWV is assessed through the calculation of the time required for a given pressure waveform to travel from a proximal to a distal site over a known distance. The AI also is clearly associated with survival. AI represents the difference between the first and second systolic peak of the pulse-wave contour divided by PP height. AI is a composite parameter because it expresses the reflective properties of the peripheral distal arterial bed and elastic properties of large arteries. Thus, these 2 measures, although correlated, are not interchangeable or synonymous. PWV and AIx are determined from contour analysis of arterial waveforms recorded by applanation tonometry (SphygmoCortm device, PWV Inc., Westmead, Sydney, Australia) using a highly reproducible technique previously described elsewhere [9, 10]. Briefly, PWV is computed from carotid and radial artery waveforms recorded consecutively (fig. 1), an ECG gated-signal simultaneously recorded, and standard anthropometrical distances ([sternal notch to arterial radial site distance] – [sternal notch to carotid site distance]), as required by the SphygmoCortm software.

PWV and AI assessed by means of applanation tonometry, a simple bedside-applicable technique, may be particularly promising in pharmacological studies dealing with the influence of different substances (mainly antihypertensive drugs) on the viscoelastic properties of large arteries [9–11].

Arterial Compliance and Hypertension

In patients with essential hypertension the arterial compliance is significantly reduced. Also in borderline hypertensives arterial distensibility is already reduced at a young age. It is still unclear whether the reduction of arterial compliance is caused by increased arterial pressure or by reduction of arterial wall dynamic properties.

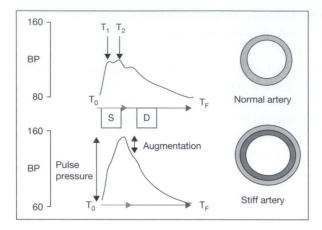

Fig. 1. Typical pulse waveforms from (top) normal and (bottom) stiffened conduit arteries derived from percutaneous tonometry tracings. With reference to a normal artery: T0 = time of start of cardiac cycle; TF = time of finish of cardiac cycle; T1 = time to outgoing pressure peak; T2 = time to peak of reflected wave; S = systole; D = diastole. Peaks at T1 and T2 coincide in the stiffened artery, leading to augmentation of arterial pressure. AI is the augmentation pressure (the difference between the second and the first systolic peak measured on the aortic pressure waveform) divided by PP (pulse-wave height) × 100 [11].

Recent studies suggest that intrinsic changes in the arterial wall produce increased stiffness in the arteries. Therefore, the treatment for hypertension must be directed not only to reduce blood pressure but to improve arterial wall compliance [12, 13].

Blood pressure includes a steady component – the mean arterial pressure, and a pulsatile component – the pulse pressure (the difference between systolic and diastolic pressure), which is the result of intermittent ventricular ejection. Pulse pressure is also influenced by the cushioning capacity of large arteries (expressed by compliance) and by the timing and intensity of waves from the heart to vessels and back to the heart (expressed by PWV). All blood vessels have a conduit function that means supplying the organs with blood and a cushioning function that implies dampening the oscillation, but larger arteries are more useful in cushioning and smaller arteries are more useful in blood distribution [14].

The cushioning function is specifically altered during hypertension.

The physiopathology of arterial rigidity includes structural and functional aspects.

High blood pressure injures the arterial wall, increases matrix collagen deposition and reduces the elastin/collagen ratio. In large arteries 50% of arterial wall is occupied by the matrix. Therefore, interstitial accumulation of collagen capable of water immobilization has a profound impact on the structure and mechanical properties of the large arteries.

In young people the primary reflected wave returns to the central aorta in diastole, where it augments coronary and cerebral perfusion. If the artery is stiff, the primary reflected wave arrives back at the aortic root during late systole, where it is superimposed on the incident wave, adding to central pulse pressure and cardiac afterload [15]. Arterial stiffness has deleterious effects on left ventricular function and increases myocardial oxygen consumption [16].

Vascular stiffness is also accompanied by changes in the left ventricle that increase end-systolic chamber stiffness. This does not require renal disease or cardiac hypertrophy to be present. This ventricular arterial stiffening alters the heart response to stress, salt overload or abrupt changes in heart function in patients with heart failure and preserved ejection fraction. The ventricular-arterial stiffness impacts on cardiovascular reserve and blood pressure lability, and also decreases diastolic blood pressure and impairs coronary perfusion [17].

Small arteries also have an important role in hypertension.

Enhanced constriction of these arteries in hypertension may increase peripheral resistance by reducing lumen diameter. According to Poiseuille's law, a small decrease in lumen size may induce significant hemodynamic change and may increase systemic vascular resistance. In small vessels, the main reproducible parameter is media-lumen ratio, measured by histologic techniques, entirely different than large arteries parameters measurement described in the previous section. Studies done on samples taken from gluteal fat confirm that small vessel remodeling does not require true hypertrophy [18]. Here, the media width is increased but the outer and inner diameters are reduced. In early hypertension this eutrophic remodeling is dominant, and only in longstanding hypertension does the well-known hypertrophic remodeling become predominant. This new view of arteriosclerosis-eutrophic remodeling is thought to apply also for large vessels, including the aorta. The 'small aorta syndrome' is more prevalent than dilated aorta in longstanding hypertension [19].

The main role in remodeling is played by the extracellular matrix. Collagen deposition is significantly enhanced in small arteries in patients with essential hypertension. Deposits of collagen contribute to media thickness. Collagen deposition is enhanced by different hormones, such as endothelin-1, angiotensin II and catecholamines. Metalloproteinase activity that degrades extracellular matrix protein is also diminished [20, 21].

Another remodeling process in hypertension is vascular rarefaction. In subjects with severe hypertension the density of arterioles is decreased, which increases vascular resistance [22].

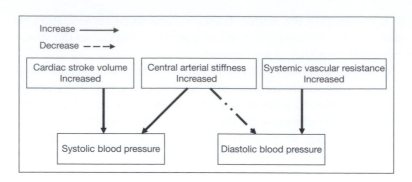

Fig. 2. Factors which influence systolic and diastolic blood pressure.

Figure 2 presents, in a concise manner, the factors that influence systolic and diastolic hypertension.

Finally, the change in permeability in the vasa vasorum network, a vascular system that originates from intercostal arteries that provides blood to the arterial wall, may have a role in arterial rigidity by impairing the clearance atherogenic factors and reducing blood wall oxygenation [23].

Arterial Compliance and Diabetes

Diabetic patients show increased arterial stiffness at a relatively young age compared with nondiabetic subjects. Also, diabetes is associated with increased ventricular stiffness in the presence of normal ventricular ejection fraction [24, 25].

Arterial compliance is affected both in insulin-dependent diabetes mellitus and non-insulin-dependent diabetes mellitus subjects from an early stage [26, 27].

This finding suggests that in diabetes the normal aging process of the arterial wall is accelerated. In diabetes, a nonenzymatic reaction between glucose and protein takes place in the arterial wall. At the beginning, glucose and proteins form an unstable and reversible product, called the Schiff base. After a period of time, days to weeks, the unstable product accumulates and forms a more stable product named the Amadori product. The best known Amadori product is hemoglobin A1C, which is glucose linked to the N-terminal valine amino group of the beta chain of hemoglobin.

If exposure to high glucose concentration is longer and hyperglycemia is not lowered, the Amadori product retransforms again into a very stable product, virtually irreversible and resistant to degradation, named 'advanced glycosylation end product' or AGE. AGEs alter arterial wall by cross linking throughout the collagen molecule, and the result is loss of compliance. In uncontrolled diabetes, the formation of AGEs is accelerated [24, 28]. Accumulation of AGEs is not an isolated phenomenon and can worsen the damage done by hypercholesterolemia, smoking and renal failure. AGEs increase low-density cholesterol trapping through covalent links. Low-density cholesterol links to collagen and elastin and worsens arterial compliance [29]. Cigarette smoking produces AGEs from tobacco, by an incompletely understood mechanism [30]. Patients with advanced renal failure cannot clear AGEs, and these low-weight molecules accumulate. Modern hemodialysis and peritoneal dialysis methods are unable to remove AGEs efficiently [24].

Recent experimental studies showed that AGE cross-link inhibitors can reverse arterial stiffness and diastolic dysfunction. Extensive presentation of this new class of experimental drugs, AGE cross-link inhibitors, is beyond the scope of this review; for an excellent overview of this issue, see Aronson [24].

The glycation end products affect both large arteries and small arteries. Large artery disease results in stroke and myocardial infarction and small artery disease predisposes to retinopathy and renal failure. Pulse pressure, PWV and AI are strong survival predictors in diabetes, independent of hypertension. Worldwide, diabetic subjects are at substantial cardiovascular risk similar to a nondiabetic subject who has sustained a myocardial infarction. More studies linking PWV to clinical outcomes of diabetes are needed to provide a better understanding of cardiovascular disease in diabetes [31–33].

Arterial Compliance, Obesity and Metabolic Syndrome

Obesity is associated with early vascular changes. Excess body fat, abdominal visceral fat and larger waist circumference have been identified as risk factors for accelerated arterial stiffening in young and older adults. Several pre-existing risk factors, including diabetes, hypertension and dyslipidemia, may particularly increase the negative cardiovascular effects of morbid obesity, causing greater cardiovascular risk earlier in adulthood. There are a number of mechanisms by which increasing adiposity and obesity might contribute to arterial stiffening, both in the short and the long term. First, the state of insulin resistance that commonly accompanies obesity impairs endothelium-dependent vasodilatation and increases the local activity of a variety of growth factors in vascular tissue, promoting collagen production and the development of vascular smooth muscle cell hypertrophy [34, 35].

In addition, the pro-inflammatory state typical of obesity may promote free radical formation, leading to the development of oxidative stress. Elevated sympathetic nerve activity and norepinephrine-evoked vascular smooth muscle cell contraction may also contribute to obesity-related stiffness [34]. Finally, obesity might increase arterial stiffness through the hormone leptin, which has been shown to promote angiogenesis and vascular smooth muscle cell proliferation [36].

Obesity is often accompanied by a metabolic syndrome, and substantial improvement of the latter also occurs with weight loss. Weight loss in obese individuals leads to rapid improvement of cardiovascular risk factors; however, some studies suggested that weight loss may be hazardous in the long term [37].

A recent study showed that dramatic weight reduction in obese patients with cardiovascular risks corrects metabolic derangements and improves small vessel compliance [34]. Endothelial dysfunction and alterations in function and structure of the arterial wall are detectable earlier in small arterioles than in larger arteries. Lack of change in large artery compliance after weight loss may imply that the process of tissue repair in the large arteries is lengthy and may take several months of stable reduced weight [38].

A metabolic syndrome is defined by the presence of hypertension in association with two or more of the following criteria: high-density lipoprotein <40 mg/dl in men and <50 mg/dl in women, fasting glucose between 100 and 125 mg/dl, triglycerides >150 mg/dl or drug treatment for elevated triglycerides, and waist circumference >102 cm in men or 88 cm in women [39]. Several studies showed that that metabolic syndrome even without diabetes increases the risk of hypertensive target organ damage [40, 41]. Moreover, arterial distensibility is reduced in nondiabetic healthy persons with insulin resistance syndrome and in patients with metabolic syndrome, indicating that arterial stiffness is an early sign of pathology in this disorder [42]. Also, stiffness increases in people with a family history of diabetes [43].

A recent study showed that a metabolic syndrome increases arterial stiffness independent of the effect of hypertension. A possible mechanism is accumulation of advanced glycation end products and enhanced oxidative stress, which alter the structure and function of collagen and elastin.

Insulin resistance, the elevation of leptin and a low level of adiponectin have an additive effect. The elevated pulse pressure in metabolic syndrome can explain the increased risk of cardiovascular morbidity associated with this disease [40].

Arterial Stiffness and Survival in Patients with Chronic Kidney Disease

In industrialized societies, there is a close relationship between hypertension and progressive impairment of renal function. Hypertension and its associated disorder, diabetes mellitus, are the principal reasons for cardiovascular disease and the initiation of renal replacement therapy with dialysis or transplantation [44]. Cardiovascular events and mortality increase as glomerular filtration rate slows down to below 60 ml/min or albuminuria is present only in a modest degree. In dialysis patients, cardiovascular disease is 10- to 20-fold higher than in the general population, representing at least half of the 15–25% per year mortality rate [45–47]. The fact that only a small minority of people with hypertension develop terminal renal failure is probably best explained by the time interval necessary for renal failure to develop; most hypertensives die of cardiovascular failure before terminal renal failure occurs.

Parameters of arterial stiffness have been associated significantly with cardiovascular morbidity and mortality in patients with essential hypertension and renal failure. Aortic stiffness is an independent predictor of primary coronary events in these patients [49, 50]. Furthermore, increased PWV and AI are strong and independent predictors of cardiovascular death in hypertensive and chronic kidney patients, even without clinically evident atherosclerosis. There is a direct association between parameters of arterial stiffness (PWV and AIx) and the worsening of coronary disease assessed by coronary angiography independent of traditional and nontraditional risk factors: age, dyslipidemia, diabetes, blood pressure, inflammatory status and calcium-phosphate metabolism [51]. Larger values of AI and PWV in terminal renal disease populations are either treated by peritoneal dialysis or hemodialysis, but patients treated by peritoneal dialysis have a worse overall prognosis. This finding is explained by poorer blood volume control and worse lipid profile in patients treated by peritoneal dialysis [52]. There are studies that suggest that in the terminal renal population, the arterial stiffness changes only after renal transplantation, but the data are relatively scarce [53].

There are several potential pathophysiological pathways that could explain why the marked reduction in large artery compliance negatively impacts cardiovascular survival in chronic kidney disease patients. First, increased arterial stiffness is strongly associated, in dialysis patients, with left ventricular hypertrophy and increased left ventricular mass, recognized risk factors for cardiovascular disease. Second, premature return of reflected arterial waves from peripheral sites leads to an elevated pulse pressure and reduces the diastolic period with negative consequences on coronary perfusion, resulting in subendocardial ischemia. Two more processes in chronic kidney disease patients have recently gained considerable attention: these are calcification, and chronic inflammation [49, 50, 54]. Coronary artery calcification has been shown to be very prevalent and extremely advanced, even when compared to nonrenal patients with severe coronary artery disease. There is a strong correlation between coronary artery calcification and aortic PWV in patients with chronic kidney disease. The second important process relates to systemic inflammation. A strong correlation between C-reactive protein and PWV/AIx was found. All these data demonstrate the role of arterial stiffness in determining the poor outcome of cardiovascular disease in patients with chronic kidney disease [48–50, 54].

Arterial Stiffness and Therapy

Several dietary modifications are efficient in reducing stiffness. Flavonoids are antioxidant substances abundant in fruit, vegetables and dark chocolate that may reduce arterial stiffness [43, 55]. Restriction of dietary sodium and reducing passive and active cigarette and cigar smoking have a beneficial effect on arterial compliance.

Moderate alcohol consumption and regular aerobic exercise (walking, jogging or swimming) may also improve arterial elasticity [43, 56].

Rapid weight loss in patients with morbid obesity and cardiovascular risk factors who underwent laparoscopic adjustable gastric banding was found to be associated with improvement of small artery compliance [34].

The clinical benefits of enhanced external counterpulsation therapy in chronic stable refractory angina patients who fail to respond to conventional therapy, like percutaneous coronary intervention or bypass surgery combined with aggressive antianginal medication, include reductions in angina episodes, nitrate use and improvement in exercise tolerance and quality of life. In a recent study, enhanced external counterpulsation treatment improved AI and PWV [57].

Interventional studies regarding the effect of drugs on arterial compliance are rare. Captopril, propranolol and amlodipine significantly reduced PWV compared with placebo, whereas verapamil had no acute effect on arterial stiffness [58, 59]. Nitroglycerin had a highly significant effect on AI, but just a minor effect on PWV, suggesting that the former parameter may be more useful in pharmacological studies [60]. Spironolactone prevents the accumulation of aortic and myocardial collagen, independent of BP changes, in spontaneously hypertensive rats. Investigations on the long-term effect of spironolactone on arterial stiffness are underway [61]. Counting the multiple effects of the rennin-angiotensin-aldosterone (RAA) axis on the endothelium, RAA inhibition seems particularly attractive in reducing arterial stiffness. Compared with a thiazide diuretic, losartan significantly improved the AI. In patients with essential hypertension, both ACE inhibition and blockade of angiotensin receptor-1 reduced arterial stiffness. Treatment with valsartan in patients with essential hypertension improved arterial compliance of both large and small vessels [62].

This effect was even more pronounced by the 'dual' blockade of the RAA system [63, 64].

Clinical studies of hypertensive humans have shown that the antistiffening effect of converting enzyme inhibition is more pronounced in the presence of the c variant of the AT1R receptor gene polymorphism. The hypertensive patients with this type of polymorphism derive more benefit from converting enzyme inhibitors than from treatment with other hypertensive drugs [65].

Omapatrilat, a combined inhibitor of ACE and neutral endopeptidase, has been shown to decrease pulse pressure and proximal aortic stiffness much more than ACE inhibitor alone. This finding indicates the possibility that inhibition of neutral endopeptidase improves aortic elastic characteristics by affecting bradykinin, natriuretic peptides and metalloproteinases [66].

Antihypertensive therapy improves arterial stiffness mainly by reducing BP as a major determinant of diminished arterial compliance. Currently used antihypertensive drugs that may potentially alter arterial stiffness involve the risk of inappropriately decreasing diastolic BP, thus jeopardizing coronary reserve. Moreover, high BP alone definitely does not determine arterial stiffness, which is also influenced by BP-independent structural modifications of the large artery walls [67]. Therapeutic studies focusing on structural improvement in the vessel walls are just beginning. Promising targets in this respect are the matrical proteins. During degenerative processes of the arterial wall, these proteins are establishing nonenzymatic links to glucose (and other similar molecules), and generating advanced glycation end products (AGEs). These AGEs accumulate slowly at the level of low-turnover proteins, such as collagen and elastin, increasing arterial (and myocardial) stiffness. Reducing AGE generation may improve arterial compliance [68]. A recent clinical trial found that a breaker of AGE (ALT-711) improves vascular distensibility and ventricular diastolic distensibility [24, 69]. Treatment with rosiglitazone has reduced hyperinsulinemia and improved small artery elasticity with a tendency to improve large artery elasticity in hypertensive as well as normotensive patients. Rosiglitazone improves insulin receptor sensitivity (IRS), a finding which supports the hypothesis that hyperinsulinemia and IRS participate in the mechanisms of tissue injury and that their improvement induces improvement in arterial elasticity [70]. Therapy with statins may also improve arterial stiffness. Recent investigations showed that PWV improved after fluvastatin and atorvastatin treatment in hypertensive patients, with or without end-stage renal failure [59, 71].

A novel approach to vascular stiffness is treatment with the PDE5a inhibitor sildenafil. Sildenafil is used to treat erectile dysfunction. In the vascular wall sildenafil increases cGMP activation and results in inhibition of fibrosis and vascular relaxation [72].

New drugs that enhance elastin by blocking neutrophil elasticity have been tried, but the study was limited by the toxicity of these drugs [73].

Renal transplantation is the preferred method of renal replacement therapy in most patients with ESRD, because renal transplantation largely restores renal function and patient's quality of life, and considerably improves survival, including CV morbidity and mortality, compared with dialysis patients [74, 75]. AI and PWV in living renal transplant recipients were significantly lower than in HD patients [75–77]. Cyclosporine A treatment, known as a possible factor of renal vasoconstriction, did not induce an acute increase in arterial stiffness by using applanation tonometry [77].

Arterial stiffness seems to have a genetic component, which is largely independent of the influence of blood pressure and other cardiovascular risk factors. Recent studies on animals and humans have looked for the structural and genetic bases of arterial stiffness. They have shown that several genes and molecules are associated with vascular wall stiffening and have illustrated the consequences of changes in these genes and molecules under various clinical conditions. There is strong evidence that arterial stiffness is affected by the amount and density of stiff wall material and the spatial organization of that material. To identify these molecules and their signaling pathways is important for the development of future drug treatments of arterial stiffness [78]. Extensive presentation of the genetic characteristic of arterial stiffness is beyond the scope of this chapter; for an excellent overview, see Laurent et al. [78].

References

1   Hayden MR, Sowers JR, Tyagi SR: The central role of vascular extracellular matrix and basement membrane remodeling in metabolic syndrome and type 2 diabetes: the matrix preloaded. Cardiovasc Diabetol 2005;4:9.
2   Siperstein MD: Diabetic microangiopathy and the control of blood glucose. N Engl J Med 1983;309:1577–1599.
3   Klein RF, Feingold KR, Morgan C, Stern WH, Siperstein MD: Relationship of muscle capillary basement membrane thickness and diabetic retinopathy. Diabetes Care 1987;10:195–199.
4   London GM, Marchais SJ, Guerin AP, et al: Arterial structure and function in end-stage renal failure. Nephrol Dial Transplant 2002;17:1713–1724.
5   O'Rouke MF, Kelly RP: Wave reflection in the systemic circulation and its implication in the ventricular function. J Hypertens 1993;11:327–337.
6   Izzo JL Jr: Hypertension in elderly: a pathophysiologic approach to therapy. J Am Geriatr Soc 1982;30:352–359.
7   Tozawa M, et al: Pulse pressure and risk of total mortality and cardiovascular events in patients on chronic hemodialysis. Kidney Int 2002;61:717–726.
8   Chadwick RS, et al: Pulse-wave model of brachial arterial pressure modulation in aging and hypertension. Am J Physiol 1986;251:H1–H11.
9   Seyrek N, et al: Which parameter is more influential on the development of arteriosclerosis in hemodialysis patients? Ren Fail 2003;25:1011–1018.
10 Mourad JJ, Pannier B, Blacher J, et al: Creatinine clearance, pulse wave velocity, carotid compliance and essential hypertension. Kidney Int 2001;59:1834–1841.
11 Covic A, et al: Arterial stiffness in renal patients: an update. Am J Kidney Dis 2005;45: 965–977.

12   Reneman RS, Meinders JM, Hoeks APG: Non-invasive ultrasound in arterial wall dynamics in humans: what have we learned and what remains to be solved. Eur Heart J 2005;26:960–966.
13   Bussy C, Boutouyrie P, Lacolley P, et al: Intrinsic stiffness of the carotid arterial wall in essential hypertensives. Hypertension 2000;35:1049–1054.
14   Blacher J, Protogerou AD, Safar ME: Large artery stiffness and antihypertensive agents. Curr Pharmaceut Design 2005;11:3317–3326.
15   Izzo JL Jr: Arterial stiffness and the systolic hypertension syndrome. Curr Opin Cardiol 2004;19: 341–352.
16   Safar ME, Blacher J, et al: Stiffness of carotid artery wall material and blood pressure in humans. Stroke 2000;3:782–790.
17   Kass DA: Ventricular arterial stiffening: integrating the pathophysiology. Hypertension 2005; 46:185.
18   Schiffrin EL: Remodeling of resistance arteries in essential hypertension and effects of anthypertensive treatment. AJH 2004;17:1192–1200.
19   Vasan RS, Larson MG, Levy D: Determinants of echocardiographic aortic root size: the Framingham Heart Study. Circulation 1995;91:734–740.
20   Schiffrin EL: Reactivity of small blood vessels in hypertension: relation with structural changes. Hypertension 1992;19(suppl II):II-1–II-9.
21   Schiffrin EL, Park JB, Intengan HD, et al: Correction of arterial structure and endothelial dysfunction in human essential hypertension by the angiotensin antagonist losartan. Circulation 2000;101:1653–1659.
22   Serne EH, Gans ROB, et al: Impaired skin capillary recruitment in essential hypertension is caused by both functional and structural capillary rarefaction. Hypertension 2000;38: 238–242.
23   Et-Taouil K, Safar M, Plante GE: Mechanisms and consequences of large artery rigidity. Can J Physiol Pharmacol 2003;81:205–211.
24   Aronson D: Cross-linking of glycated collagen in the pathogenesis of arterial and myocardial stiffening of aging and diabetes. J Hypertens 2003;21:3–12.
25   Lehmann ED, Riley WA, et al: Non-invasive assessment of cardiovascular disease in diabetes mellitus. Lancet 1997;350:SI14–SI19.
26   Riggs TW, Transue D: Doppler echocardiographic evaluation of left ventricular diastolic function in adolescents with diabetes mellitus. Am J Cardiol 1990;65:899–902.
27   Poirier P, Bogaty P, et al: Diastolic dysfunction in normotensive men with well-controlled type 2 diabetes: importance in maneuvers in echocardiographic screening for preclinical diabetic cardiomyopathy. Diabetes Care 2001;24:5–10.
28   Brownlee M, Cerami A, Vlassara H: Advanced glycosilation end products in tissue and the biochemical basis of diabetic complications. N Engl J Med 1988;318:1315–1321.
29   Ferrier KE, Muhlmann MH, et al: Intensive cholesterol reduction lowers blood pressure and large arterial stiffness in isolated systolic hypertension. J Am Coll Cardiol 2002;39:1020–1025.
30   Liang Yl, Shiel LM, et al: Effects of blood pressure, smoking and their interaction on carotid artery structure and function. Hypertension 2001;37:6–11.
31   Jennings GLR, Kingwell BA: Measuring arterial function in diabetes. J Hypertens 2004;22: 1863–1865.
32   Lacy PS, O'Brien DG, et al: Increased pulse wave velocity is not associated with elevated augmentation index in patients with diabetes. J Hypertens 2004;22:1937–1944.
33   Lim HS, Lip GYH: Arterial stiffness in diabetes and hypertension. J Hum Hypertens 2004;18: 467–468.
34   Shargorodsky M, Fleed A, Boaz M, Gavish D, Zimlichman R: The effect of a rapid weight loss induced by laparoscopic adjustable gastric banding on arterial stiffness, metabolic and inflammatory parameters in patients with morbid obesity. Int J Obes 2006;30:1632–1638.
35   Montagni M, Quon MJ: Insulin action in vascular endothelium: potential mechanisms linking insulin resistance with hypertension. Diabetes Obes Metab 2000;2:285–292.
36   Rizzoni D, Porteri E, et al: Structural alterations in subcutaneous small arteries of normotensive and hypertensive patients with non-insulin-dependent diabetes mellitus. Circulation 2001;103: 1238–1244.

37   Sorensen TIA, Rissansen A, et al: Intention to lose weight, weight changes, and 18-year mortality in overweight individuals without co-morbidities. Plos Med 2005;2:e171.

38   Grey E, Bratelli C, et al: Reduced small artery but not large artery elasticity is an independent risk marker for cardiovascular events. Am J Hypertens 2003;16:265–269.

39   Grundy SM, Cleeman JI, Daniels SR, et al: Diagnosis and management of the metabolic syndrome: an American Heart Association/National Heart, Lung and Blood Institute scientific statement. Curr Opin Cardiol 2006;21:1–6.

40   Mule G, Nardi E, Cottone S, et al: Relationship of metabolic syndrome with pulse pressure in patients with essential hypertension. AJH 2007;20:197–203.

41   Mule G, Nardi E, Cottone S, et al: Influence of metabolic syndrome on hypertension-related target organ damage. J Intern Med 2005;257:503–513.

42   Van Popele NM, Westendorp ICD, Bots ML, et al: Variables of the insulin resistance syndrome are associated with reduced arterial distensibility in healthy non-diabetic middle-aged women. Diabetologia 2000;43:665–672.

43   Vlachopoulos C, Aznaouridis K, Stefanidis C: Clinical appraisal of arterial stiffness: the Argonauts in front of the Golden Fleece. Heart 2006;92:1544–1550.

44   Keith DS, Nichols GA, Gullion CM, et al: Longitudinal follow-up and outcomes among a population with chronic kidney disease in a large managed care organization. Arch Intern Med 2004;164:659–663.

45   Lowrie EG, Lew NL: Death risk in hemodialysis patients: the predictive value of commonly measured variables and an evaluation of death rate differences between facilities. Am J Kidney Dis 1990;15:458–482.

46   Go AS, Chertow GM, Fan D, et al: Chronic kidney disease and the risks of death, cardiovascular events and hospitalization. N Engl J Med 2004;351:1296–1305.

47   Covic A, Mardare N, Gusbech-Tatomir P, et al: Arterial wave reflections and mortality in hemodialysis patients – only relevant in elderly, cardiovascularly compromised? Nephrol Dial Transplant 2006;21:2859–2866.

48   Goldsmith DJ, Ritz E, Covic A: Vascular calcification – a stiff challenge for the nephrologist: does preventing bone disease cause arterial disease? Kidney Int 2004;66:1315–1333.

49   Goodman WG, Goldin J, et al: Coronary-artery calcification in young adults with end-stage renal disease who are undergoing dialysis. N Engl J Med 2000;342:1478–1483.

50   Chertow GM, et al: Sevelamer attenuates the progression of coronary and aortic calcification in hemodialysis patients. Kidney Int 2002;62:245–252.

51   He ZX, Hedrick TD, et al: Severity of artery calcification by EBCT predicts silent myocardial ischemia. Circulation 2000;101:244–251.

52   Winkelmayer WC, Glynn RJ, Mittleman MA, et al: Comparing mortality of elderly patients on hemodialysis versus peritoneal dialysis: a propensity score approach. J Am Soc Nephrol 2002;13:2353–2362.

53   Covic A, Goldsmith DJ, Gusbeceth-Tatomir P, et al: Successful renal transplantation decreases aortic stiffness and increases vascular reactivity in dialysis patients. Transplantation 2003;76:1573–1577.

54   Hujairi NM, Afzali B, Goldsmith DJ: Cardiac calcification in renal patients: what we do and don't know. Am J Kidney Dis 2004;43:234–243.

55   Teede HJ, McGrafth BP, DeSilva L, et al: Isoflavones reduce arterial stiffness: a placebo-controlled study in men and postmenopausal women. Arterioscler Thromb Vasc Biol 2003;23:1066–1071.

56   Vlachopoulos C, Aznaouridis K, et al: Effect of dark chocolate on arterial function in healthy individuals. Am J Hypertens 2005;18:785–791.

57   Nichols WW, Estrada JC, Braith RW, et al: Enhanced external counterpulsation treatment improves arterial wall properties and wave reflection characteristics in patients with refractory angina. J Am Coll Cardiol 2006;48:1208–1214.

58   Kahonen M, Ylitalo R, Koobi T, et al: Influence of captopril, propranolol, and verapamil on arterial pulse wave velocity and other cardiovascular parameters in healthy volunteers. Int J Clin Pharmacol Ther 1998;36:483–489.

59   Leibovitz E, Beniashvili M, Zimlichman R, Freiman A, Shargorodsky M, Gavish D: Treatment with amlodipine and atorvastatin have additive effect in improvement of arterial compliance in hypertensive hyperlipidemic patients. Am J Hypertens 2003;16:715–718.

60 Kelly RP, Millasseau SC, Ritter JM, et al: Vasoactive drugs influence aortic augmentation index independently of pulse-wave velocity in healthy men. Hypertension 2001;37:1429–1433.
61 Safar ME, Avolio A: Aldosterone antagonism and arterial stiffness. Hypertension 2004;43:e3.
62 Shargorodsky M, Leibovitz E, Lubimov L, Gavish D, Zimlichman R: Prolonged treatment with the AT1 receptor blocker, valsartan, increases small and large artery compliance in uncomplicated essential hypertension. Am J Hypertens 2002;15:1087–1091.
63 Mahmud A, Feely J: Effect of angiotensin II receptor blockade on arterial stiffness: beyond blood pressure reduction. Am J Hypertens 2002;15:1092–1095.
64 Mahmud A, Feely J: Reduction in arterial stiffness with angiotensin II antagonist is comparable with and additive to ACE inhibition. Am J Hypertens 2002;15:321–325.
65 Benetos A, Cambien F, Gautier S: Influence of the angiotensin type 1receptor gene polymorphism on the effects of perindopril and nitrendipine on arterial stiffness in hypertensive individuals. Hypertension 1996;28:1081–1084.
66 Mitchell GF, Izzo JL Jr, et al: Omapatrilat reduces pulse pressure and proximal aortic stiffness in patients with systolic hypertension: results of the conduit hemodynamics of omapatrilat international research study. Circulation 2002;105:2955–2961.
67 Safar ME: Epidemiological findings imply that goals for drug treatment of hypertension need to be revised. Circulation 2001;103:1188–1190.
68 Kass DA, Shapiro EP, Kawaguchi M, et al: Improved arterial compliance by a novel advanced glycation end product crosslink breaker. Circulation 2001;104:1464–1470.
69 Kass DA: Ventricular arterial stiffening: integrating the pathophysiology. Hypertension 2005;46:185.
70 Shargorodsky M, Wainstein J, Gavish D, Leibovitz E, Matas Z, Zimlichman R: Treatment with rosiglitazone reduces hyperinsulinemia and improves arterial elasticity in patients with type 2 diabetes mellitus. Am J Hypertens 2003;16:617–622.
71 Ichihara A, Hayashi M, Ryuzaki M, et al: Fluvastatin prevents development of arterial stiffness in hemodialysis patients with type 2 diabetes mellitus. Nephrol Dial Transplant 2002;17:1513–1517.
72 Ohta K, Nakajima T, et al: Elafin-overexpressing mice have improved cardiac function after myocardial infarction. Am J Physiol 2004;287:H286–H292.
73 Vlachopoulos C, Hirata K, O'Rouke MF: Effect of sildenafil on arterial stiffness and wave reflection. Vasc Med 2003;8:243–248.
74 Aakhus S, Dahl K, Widerøe TE: Cardiovascular morbidity and risk factors in renal transplant patients. Nephrol Dial Transplant 1999;14:648–654.
75 Ferro CJ, Savage T, Pinder SJ, et al: Central aortic pressure augmentation in stable renal transplant recipients. Kidney Int 2002;62:166–171.
76 Covic A, Goldsmith DJ, Gusbeth-Tatomir P, et al: Successful renal transplantation decreases aortic stiffness and increases vascular reactivity in dialysis patients. Transplantation 2003;76:1573–1577.
77 Zoungas S, Kerr PG, Chadban S, et al: Arterial function after successful renal transplantation. Kidney Int 2004;65:1882–1889.
78 Laurent S, Boutuyrie P, Lacolley P: Structural and genetic bases of arterial stiffness. Hypertension 2005;45:1050.

Prof. Reuven Zimlichman
Chief of Medicine, Wolfson Medical Center
POB 5
Holon 58100 (Israel)
Tel. +972 3 502 8614, Fax +972 3 503 2693, E-Mail zimlich@post.tau.ac.il

Fisman EZ, Tenenbaum A (eds): Cardiovascular Diabetology: Clinical, Metabolic and Inflammatory
Facets. Adv Cardiol. Basel, Karger, 2008, vol 45, pp 82–106

Hypertension and Diabetes

Ehud Grossman[a]   *Franz H. Messerli*[b]

[a]Department of Internal Medicine D and Hypertension Unit, The Chaim Sheba
Medical Center, Tel-Hashomer, Israel; [b]Luke's-Roosevelt Hospital and Columbia
University, New York, N.Y., USA

Abstract

Both essential hypertension and diabetes mellitus affect the same major target organs.
The common denominator of hypertensive/diabetic target organ-disease is the vascular tree.
Left ventricular hypertrophy and coronary artery disease are much more common in diabetic
hypertensive patients than in patients suffering from hypertension or diabetes alone. The combined presence of hypertension and diabetes concomitantly accelerates the decrease in renal
function, the development of diabetic retinopathy and the development of cerebral diseases.
Lowering blood pressure to less than 130/80 mm Hg is the primary goal in the management of
the hypertensive diabetic patients. Beta-blockers have been reported to adversely affect the
overall risk factor profile in the diabetic patient. In contrast, calcium antagonists, angiotensin-
converting enzyme inhibitors and angiotensin receptor blockers have been reported to be either
neutral or beneficial with regard to the overall metabolic risk factor profile. Combination therapy is usually required to achieve blood pressure goal in diabetic patients. The addition of
aldosterone antagonists may be beneficial in patients with resistant hypertension and low levels
of serum potassium. Aggressive control of blood pressure, cholesterol and glucose levels
should be attempted to reduce the cardiovascular risk of diabetic hypertensive patients.

Introduction

The tide of diabetes is rising in the United States and all over the globe,
thereby becoming an increasingly powerful threat to global health. In the
United States alone, the prevalence of diabetes has doubled from 1990 to the
year 2000. The World Health Organization projects that by the year 2025 more
than 5% of the world population, i.e. 300 million people will suffer from diabetes. A patient who suffers from type 2 diabetes has a 2–4 times greater risk of
death from cardiovascular causes than the patient without diabetes [1]. The most

common cause of dying in the diabetic patient is heart disease. In addition, peripheral vascular disease, end-stage renal disease, blindness and amputations are common co-morbidities in diabetic patients.

Hypertension has been identified as a major risk factor for the development of diabetes. Patients with hypertension are at a 2–3 times higher risk of developing diabetes than patients with normal blood pressure [2]. Hypertension by itself is, of course, a powerful risk factor for cardiovascular morbidity and mortality as established by data from the Framingham cohort more than three decades ago. For any given level of systolic blood pressure, the occurrence of diabetes distinctly increases cardiovascular mortality. Stamler et al. [3] have documented that diabetes in the normotensive patient confers greater risk than a systolic blood pressure between 160 and 170 mm Hg. This observation provoked Haffner and Cassells' [4] observation that the prognosis of diabetes is just as grim as the one of a patient who has suffered an acute myocardial infarction. Of note, while this is true for overall cardiovascular mortality, it does not necessarily mean that diabetes and hypertension are synonymous in affecting the individual components of cardiovascular system. Also, it does by no means follow that specific cardiovascular drugs are equally protective in diabetes and coronary artery disease.

Blood pressure control remains unacceptably low in the general population, but is even lower in the diabetic hypertensive patient [5]. Although controlling the blood pressure is a commendable goal of antihypertensive therapy, treating hypertensive cardiovascular disease in the diabetic patient is more complex than simply achieving blood pressure targets. Recent studies have shown that antihypertensive drug classes have differing effects on the risk of new onset diabetes, on metabolic endocrine surrogate endpoints and possibly on outcome [6]. The present chapter reviews the epidemiology of hypertension and diabetes and discusses clinical findings and gives some recommendations for therapy of the diabetic hypertensive patient.

Epidemiology

Between 1976 and 1988, the prevalence of diabetes (among people age 40–74 years) rose from 11.4 to 14.3% in the USA [7]. Similar increase in the prevalence of diabetes has been described in other parts of the world [8–10]. It is estimated that globally, the number of people with diabetes will rise from 151 millions in the year 2000 to 221 million by the year 2010 and to 300 million by 2025 [11].

The projections of increasing numbers of people with diabetes are driven mainly by the anticipated world population growth, especially amongst the middle-aged and elderly. This spectacular increase in the frequency of type 2 diabetes is being paralleled by a similar alarming increase in obesity [12] which is the major risk factor for type 2 diabetes. Improved nutrition, better hygiene and control of many communicable diseases, have increased longevity. In addition, life-style changes that have been well documented in some countries [13] and include higher fat diets and decreased physical activity contributed to the increase prevalence of type 2 diabetes. The rising prevalence of obesity and type 2 diabetes is also observed in children and is yet another symptom of the effects of globalization and industrialization, with sedentary lifestyle and obesity as the predominant factors involved. Recently, other categories of abnormal glucose metabolism that are not defined as overt diabetes, such as impaired glucose tolerance (IGT) and impaired fasting glucose (IGF), were introduced. These two conditions also carry a higher risk of future diabetes and probably also of cardiovascular disease [14]. The prevalence of these categories is also increasing and in a recent study the prevalence of IGT in an Australian population was as high as 10.6% [15]. Type 2 diabetes is a descriptive term and a manifestation of a much broader underlying disorder. This includes metabolic syndrome, a cluster of cardiovascular risk factors which apart from glucose intolerance includes hyperinsulinemia, dislipidemia, hypertension, visceral obesity, hypercoagulability and microalbuminuria [16]. This combination of risk factors is partly responsible for the increased risk of cardiovascular disease in diabetes [16].

The prevalence of hypertension is expected to increase in the next 25 years from 26.5% in the year 2000 to 29.2% in the year 2025 [17]. The incidence of hypertension in patients with type 2 diabetes is approximately twofold higher than in age-matched subjects without the disease [18]. The definition of hypertension is different in diabetes, and blood pressure levels above 130/80 mm Hg are already defined as hypertension in diabetic patients [19]. The prevalence of hypertension is particularly high in obese subjects and it increases with age. The pattern of hypertension is changes as patients get older. The systolic blood pressure increases linearly with age across all age ranges, whereas diastolic blood pressure increases with age only until the age of 50 and then levels off and declines. Thus, in the elderly isolated systolic hypertension is more common [20]. Since the prevalence of type 2 diabetes is high in obese subjects and it increases with age, the co-existence of diabetes and hypertension is particularly high in obese and/or elderly patients.

Diabetic patients have more isolated systolic hypertension, and due to autonomic neuropathy they experience less nocturnal fall in blood pressure and higher baseline heart rate than their nondiabetic counterparts [5].

The co-existence of diabetes and hypertension in the same patient is devastating to the cardiovascular system [1, 21] and blood pressure control in these patients is a great challenge, since the target blood pressure is lower and the response to treatment is poor [5].

Clinical Findings

Diabetes mellitus is associated with a high risk of cardiovascular disease and is the leading cause of end-stage renal disease, blindness, and nontraumatic amputations in western countries [18]. Elevated but nondiabetic levels of fasting glucose also carry a higher risk of cardiovascular disease [14]. As a cardiovascular risk factor, glycemia is a continuous variable with no sudden increase in risk [22]. The extreme state is the metabolic syndrome that is associated with a 2- to 3-fold increase in cardiovascular morbidity and mortality [23–25]. Hypertension by itself is a powerful risk factor for cardiovascular morbidity and mortality.

Although the effects of diabetes mellitus and hypertension on the cardiovascular system vary somewhat and are often distinct, their combined presence in the same patient is destructive [26]. The common denominator of hypertensive/diabetic target organ disease is the vascular tree, which is affected by both disorders.

The Vascular Tree

Both hypertension and diabetes are well-identified risk factors for atherogenesis. Several mechanisms acting together mediate the damage to the vascular tree in the diabetic hypertensive patient [26]. Metabolic abnormalities that often present in diabetic hypertensive patients accelerate atherosclerosis. Plasma levels of lipoprotein have been noted to be elevated in diabetic individuals, particularly those with poor glycemic control. Augmented oxidation of low-density lipoprotein cholesterol and formation of glycated low-density lipoprotein, which enhance foam cell formation, have been observed in diabetic states. Anatomic and functional abnormalities of the vascular endothelium have been described in diabetes mellitus and hypertension [26].

Hyperglycemia activates protein kinase C in endothelial cells, which may enhance vascular tone, permeability, and atherosclerosis. Elevated circulating levels of insulin as exist in type 2 diabetes and in many patients with essential hypertension may contribute either directly or in conjunction with insulin-like growth factor (IGF) to the accelerated atherosclerosis associated with these conditions. Insulin and IGF-1 may exert their atherogenic effects through influences on both vascular endothelial cells and vascular smooth muscle cells [26]. Diabetes mellitus and hypertension are also associated with hematologic abnormalities that encourage thrombosis. Enhanced platelet adhesion and aggregation as well as higher than normal levels of some coagulation factors contribute to the procoagulation state in diabetic hypertensive patients [26]. Diabetes seems to be a specific risk factor for small vessel disease. In contrast, hypertension, at least in its nonmalignant form, seems to affect predominantly the large arteries. Together, the two disorders synergistically damage the arterial tree.

The Heart

Coronary Artery Disease

Diabetes mellitus is associated with a markedly increased prevalence of coronary artery disease. The prevalence of coronary artery disease as assessed by various diagnostic methods is as high as 55% among adult patients with diabetes mellitus as compared to 2–4% of the general population [27]. Moreover, the cardiovascular mortality rate is more than doubled in men and more than quadrupled in women who have diabetes mellitus compared to those without. The restenosis rate after coronary balloon angioplasty is about 2-fold higher in diabetic than nondiabetic patients [28]. Due to autonomic neuropathy diabetic patients have a decreased perception of ischemic pain, which contributes to a high prevalence of silent ischemia [29]. Diabetic patients without previous myocardial infarction have as high a risk of myocardial infarction as nondiabetic patients with previous myocardial infarction [30].

Myocardial ischemia is common in patients with hypertension [31] and caused by several pathogenic mechanisms. (1) Hypertension accelerates arteriosclerosis of the coronary arteries. (2) Elevated blood pressure increases left ventricular wall stress, wall tension, and stroke work. (3) Resistance of the coronary microvasculature is abnormally elevated in hypertensive patients even in the absence of left ventricular hypertrophy. (4) Long-standing hypertension causes left ventricular hypertrophy that increases the diffusion distance, compromises the vasodilator reserve of the coronary circulation and increases the oxygen demand of the myocardium [1, 32]. It should be noted that hypertensive patients, especially those with left ventricular hypertrophy, are as susceptible to silent myocardial ischemia as patients with diabetes [33].

Coronary artery disease is much more common in diabetic hypertensive patients than in patients suffering from hypertension or diabetes alone [34]. For all 2,681 men in the PROCAM trial who had none of the three risk factors (i.e. hypertension, diabetes, or hyperlipidemia), the coronary artery disease incidence was 6/1,000 in 4 years. In contrast, the incidence of coronary artery disease in those participants who were suffering from hypertension or diabetes was 14 and 15 per 1,000 in 4 years, respectively. When both risk factors were present in the same patient, the incidence rate increased to 48 per 1,000 [34]. Diabetes, and to a lesser extent hypertension, may alter the perception of ischemic pain, leading to a high prevalence of silent ischemia. Melina et al. [35] found a high prevalence of asymptomatic ST segment depression in diabetic patients with essential hypertension. The number of ST segment depression episodes was significantly related to glycosylated hemoglobin levels, left ventricular mass, and ambulatory systolic and diastolic blood pressure variability and hypertensive peaks.

Cardiomyopathy

Several clinical studies have indicated that diabetes mellitus is associated with cardiomyopathy that is independent of atherosclerotic coronary artery disease [36]. Macroscopic changes include muscular hypertrophy with pale appearance and firmness to palpation. Microscopic changes include thickening of the capillary basement membrane, intimal proliferation of small myocardial arterioles and capillary microaneurysms, and focal myocardial fibrosis with an accumulation of interstitial glycoproteinand collagen. Electron microscopy shows perivascular damage with loss of contractile myocardial elements and deposition of either glycoprotein or material that is positive on periodic acid-Schiff stain [1]. Structural changes are associated with impaired ventricular function. Diastolic dysfunction is an early abnormality in diabetic cardiomyopathy and can be diagnosed even in young insulin-dependent diabetic subjects before the onset of systolic dysfunction [37]. Shapiro [38] found abnormal diastolic function in patients with diabetes mellitus who did not have heart disease. Diabetes mellitus seems to have less effect on systolic function [39]. Mustonen et al. [40] found similar resting ejection fraction in diabetic patients and controls. However, during 4 years of follow-up, the left ventricular ejection fraction at rest markedly decreased in diabetic patients only. Several studies have shown that ejection fractions after myocardial infarction are lower in diabetic than in nondiabetic patients [41]. Impaired myocardial systolic and diastolic functions may lead to congestive heart failure. Congestive heart failure is substantially increased in diabetic patients irrespective of coronary artery disease and hypertension [42]. Diabetic patients with coronary artery disease develop more severe congestive heart failure, more hospitalizations and higher risk of mortality than nondiabetic patients [43]. In the SOLVD (Studies of Left Ventricular Dysfunction) trial diabetes was an independent risk factor for morbidity and mortality in heart failure [44]. The negative impact of diabetes on symptoms and prognosis was more pronounced in women [44]. The Framingham study data revealed a fourfold greater incidence of congestive heart failure in diabetic men and an eightfold increase in diabetic women, compared with nondiabetic subjects [45]. In the DIGAMI (Diabetes Mellitus Insulin-Glucose Infusion in Acute Myocardial Infarction) trial congestive heart failure accounted for up to 66% of mortality during the first year after myocardial infarction in diabetic patients [46]. In a recent study even impaired glucose tolerance, when associated with moderate systolic hypertension, increased the risk of 8-year cardiovascular mortality in men twofold possibly through the presence of the metabolic syndrome [47]. Marroquin et al. [48] followed for 4 years 755 women from the Women's Ischemia Syndrome Evaluation (WISE) study who were referred for coronary angiography to evaluate suspected myocardial ischemia. Compared with women with normal metabolic status, women with the metabolic syndrome had a significantly lower 4-year survival rate (94.3 vs. 97.8%, p = 0.03) and event-free survival from major adverse cardiovascular events (death, nonfatal myocardial infarction, stroke, or congestive heart failure; 87.8 vs. 93.5%, p = 0.003). The higher risk was evident only in women with angiographically significant coronary artery disease.

Longstanding hypertension leads to left ventricular hypertrophy that may be either concentric or eccentric. Hemodynamic factors explain the increased left ventricular mass; however, clinical blood pressure levels are only weakly related to left ventricular mass [49].

Therefore, nonhemodynamic factors such as sodium intake, activity of growth-promoting hormones (such as insulin and thyroxin), activity of the sympathetic nervous system, rennin-angiotensin system, whole-blood viscosity glucose levels, and genetics probably contribute to the development of left ventricular hypertrophy [1]. Cardiac hypertrophy is not a homogenous process, and growth of nonmyocytic cells, which include endothelial cells, vascular smooth muscle cells, fibroblasts and macrophages participate in the development of left ventricular hypertrophy [50]. In animal models, isoenzymatic changes of cardiac myosin have been described in experimental hypertensive cardiomyopathy [51].

Hypertensive cardiomyopathy is associated with impaired cardiac function [1]. We showed that in hypertensive patients contractility deteriorated as left ventricular mass increased [52]. In early hypertensive heart disease, impaired filling is predominantly caused by decreased ventricular relaxation during early diastole [53]. Patients may have reduced exercise capacity because the stiff left ventricles are unable to accommodate the increased blood volume [54–56]. A progressive decline in ventricular function may lead to congestive heart failure. Data from the Framingham study showed that hypertension was the primary cause of congestive heart failure in 35% of the cases and played a role in this condition in another 40% [57]. In a recent survey conducted in Israel, 75% of patients with congestive heart failure had hypertension and the rate was even higher in those with diastolic dysfunction [58, 59]. The risk to develop congestive heart failure increased by 55% for a 20 mm Hg increase in systolic pressure [60] and was approximately eight times greater when electrocardiographic criteria of left ventricular hypertrophy were present [61].

The coexistence of diabetes and hypertension results in more severe cardiomyopathy than would be expected with either hypertension or diabetes mellitus alone [62]. The extensive degenerative changes in the diabetic hypertensive heart may be related to abnormalities in the microcirculation. The most striking microscopic findings of the hypertensive diabetic heart seem to be the distribution of dense interstitial connective tissue throughout the myocardium [1]. Clinical studies with echocardiography also showed an increased left ventricular mass in diabetic hypertensive patients [63, 64]. Grossman et al. [63] found increased septal and posterior wall thickness in patients with hypertension and diabetes compared with nondiabetic hypertensive patients. Prevalence of left ventricular hypertrophy was 72% in diabetic hypertensive patients and only 32% in the nondiabetic hypertensive patients who had a similar degree of hypertension. Because left ventricular hypertrophy is known to predispose patients with hypertension to cardiovascular morbid and fatal events, the finding of a high prevalence of left ventricular hypertrophy in diabetic hypertensives may partially explain the increased morbidity and mortality in these patients. Cardiomyopathy of diabetes and hypertension is associated with impaired ventricular function and a high prevalence of congestive heart failure [65].

The Kidneys

The most common causes for end-stage renal disease (ESRD) are diabetes mellitus and hypertension [66]. Patients with diabetes mellitus can develop kidney disease and about one-third develop diabetic nephropathy, which accounts for almost half of all new ESRD cases [66]. Early in the course of diabetic nephropathy, changes in kidney hemodynamics and hyperfiltration lead to an increase in glomerular filtration rate (GFR) [67]. The progression of nephropathy involves characteristic pathologic changes, including accumulation of the extracellular matrix, widening of the glomerular basement membrane, arteriosclerosis, and some degree of interstitial fibrosis [66]. The earliest clinical manifestation of diabetic nephropathy is microalbuminuria (20–200 μg/min) which, if left untreated, can progress to overt nephropathy after 10–15 years of diabetes, and is also a marker for cardiovascular disease [68, 69]. In African-Americans, albuminuria may be present in 30–40% of patients with diabetic nephropathy [66].

Hypertension is a well-defined risk factor for ESRD, and accounts for 27% of all ESRD cases in the US and 33.4% of ESRD cases among African-Americans [66]. The risk of ESRD increases as blood pressure increases [70, 71]. Analysis of the data collected from 332,544 men over a 16-year period in the MRFIT study showed that the adjusted relative risk of developing ESRD was 1.9 for high-normal blood pressure, and 22.1 for stage 4 hypertension (according to the JNC 5 criteria), relative to the category of optimal blood pressure [71]. Longstanding hypertension causes arteriolar nephrosclerosis with impaired kidney function. When hypertension is superimposed on diabetes mellitus it accelerates the decrease in renal function. Blood pressure control with levels below 130/80 mm Hg can slow the progression of renal disease in diabetic patients [72].

Peripheral Arterial Disease

In patients with type 2 diabetes mellitus peripheral arterial disease (PAD) is a major culprit for the diabetic foot. Epidemiological evidence confirms an association between diabetes and increased prevalence of PAD [73]. Individuals with diabetes have a 2- to 4-fold increase in the rate of PAD [74], more often have femoral bruits and absent pedal pulses [75], and have rates of abnormal ankle-brachial indices ranging from 11.9 to 16% [76, 77]. The duration and severity of diabetes correlate with the incidence and extent of PAD [78]. Diabetes changes the nature of PAD. Diabetic patients more commonly have infrapopliteal arterial occlusive disease and vascular calcification than non-diabetic cohorts [79]. In the Hoorn study [80], the prevalence of abnormal ankle to brachial indices was 7% in individuals with normal glucose tolerance and 20.9% in those requiring multiple hypoglycemic medications. Patients with diabetes more commonly develop the symptomatic forms of PAD, intermittent claudication, and amputation [81]. In the Framingham cohort, the presence of diabetes increased the risk of claudication by 3.5-fold in men and 8.6-fold in women. Diabetes causes most nontraumatic lower extremity amputations in the US [73].

Age, smoking and hypertension are important risk factors to develop PAD [82]. PAD presents the early clinical signs of atherosclerosis and is strongly associated with cardiovascular death [78]. Diabetic patients should be screened for PAD either by asking for symptoms and signs or taking medical history for intermittent claudication or by measuring the ankle brachial index (the ratio of ankle systolic pressure to arm systolic pressure).

Indeed, there is inadequate information regarding the role of medical therapies in diabetic patients with PAD. However, patients with diabetes should be managed by strategies of proven benefit such as smoking cessation, blood pressure control, and cholesterol control [73]. Two noninvasive therapies have demonstrated a benefit in improving walking distance in patients with PAD: exercise and cilostazol [73]. Revascularization is frequently needed in diabetic patients with PAD. In general, in patients with severe claudication or critical limb ischemia, surgery is probably superior to percutaneous transluminal angioplasty for revascularization in the femoral, popliteal, and infrapopliteal vessels but comes at a price of increased periprocedural cardiovascular morbidity and mortality [83].

The Brain

Diabetes mellitus adversely affects cerebrovascular arterial circulation. Patients with diabetes have more extracranial atherosclerosis [84]. The prevalence of diabetes among patients presenting with stroke is 3 times higher than that of matched controls [85]. In a survey conducted recently in Israel, 40% of the patients hospitalized with acute stroke had diabetes mellitus [86]. The risk of stroke is increased 150–400% for patients with diabetes [87, 88], and worsening glycemic control relates directly to stroke risk. In the Multiple Risk Factor Intervention Trial, subjects taking medications for diabetes were 3 times as likely to suffer a stroke [89]. Diabetes particularly increases the risk of stroke among younger patients [90]. The prevalence of diabetes increases the risk of stroke-related dementia more than 3-fold [91], doubles the risk of recurrence [92], and increases total and stroke-related mortality [93].

Hypertension, mainly systolic, is strongly and directly related to stroke in all age groups [94, 95] and lowering blood pressure reduces the rate of stroke remarkably [95]. The occurrence of diabetes more than doubles the risk of stroke in hypertensive patients [21] and lowering blood pressure in these patients reduces the risk of stroke by 44% [96].

The Retina

Ever since the pioneering observations of Keith, Wagener, and Barker, hypertension has been known to affect the retina. Hypertensive retinopathy consists of narrowing of the retinal arteries, dilatation of the vein crossing phenomena, and in severe cases, papilledema, cotton-wool exudates, as well as star figure in the macula. In contrast to hypertensive retinopathy, diabetic retinopathy is characterized by vascular proliferation leading to neovascularization and formation of microaneurysms.

Hypertension accelerates the development of diabetic retinopathy. Knowler et al. [97] found that in diabetic subjects not taking insulin, the incidence of exudates in those with systolic blood pressure of >145 mm Hg was more than twice that of those with pressures of <125 mm Hg. The combination of hypertension and diabetic retinopathy is often devastating and remains one of the leading causes of blindness.

Therapy

Lower Blood Pressure Target Levels

The definition of hypertension (and diabetes) is arbitrary. Hypertension is perhaps best defined as any blood pressure level that has a negative impact on the cardiovascular system. Thus, numerical definitions, although hotly debated by numerous guideline committees, are not helpful to practicing physicians. Recent guidelines set the target level of blood pressure for uncomplicated hypertension to below 140/90 mm Hg, and in the diabetic hypertensive patient to below 130/80 mm Hg [20, 24]. There is solid evidence that the benefits of blood pressure lowering are much more pronounced in the diabetic than in the nondiabetic hypertensive patient. A perhaps more physiologic way of looking at the impact of blood pressure in the diabetic hypertensive is microalbuminuria/proteinuria which is a surrogate endpoint for hypertensive renal disease and endothelial dysfunction. As long as there is significant proteinuria, a given patient's blood pressure must be considered too high for the kidneys and vascular tree. Nevertheless, the INVEST study [98] has put forward solid data that in patients with coronary artery disease (which is common in diabetic hypertensive patients) an excessive decrease in diastolic pressure may increase the risk of acute myocardial infarction. Once diastolic pressure fell below 70 mm Hg, the rate of heart attack doubled and below 60 mm Hg it tripled in this study. This would indicate that indiscriminate lowering of diastolic pressure should be avoided in patients with coronary artery disease. If such a patient has proteinuria, clinicians may find themselves in the rather puzzling situation that one target organ (the kidney) is requesting a blood pressure that the other target organ (the heart) cannot afford. This dilemma further illustrates the complexity of treatment in the diabetic hypertensive patient. Thus, the goal of lowering the blood pressure to below 130/80 mm Hg is certainly commendable, but should be considered as an appropriate target for most but not all patients.

Nonpharmacologic Therapy

Nonpharmacologic therapy, such as weight loss, low sodium diet, regular exercise, etc., has beneficial effects in hypertension, diabetes, and possibly also in patients who have both these disorders [24]. However, there is no good outcome study showing that, indeed, diet per se will decrease morbidity and mortality. Also, we should remember the paper of Sjostrom et al. [99] in obese hypertensive diabetic patients who were followed for 10 years after bariatric surgery. After a weight loss of an average of 16% which was maintained for this time period, the risk of diabetes was drastically reduced. However, although blood pressure was falling immediately after the intervention and remained low for months, the follow-up of 10 years documented no antihypertensive efficacy. Despite a weight loss of more than 20 kg, blood pressure of these patients was gradually returning to pretreatment levels. Thus, some uncertainties remain pertaining to the long-term efficacy of nonpharmacologic therapy.

The diabetic hypertensive patient is by definition a high-risk patient. The recent VALUE study [100] taught us that in such patients swift blood pressure control (within months) significantly reduces cardiovascular event rates. There is, therefore, no reason to start out with nonpharmacologic therapy alone, but we should initiate and reinforce aggressive drug therapy at the earliest possible opportunity. Counseling pertaining to diet, lifestyle and exercise can be done concomitantly or even later. Once blood pressure, lipids and glycemia are brought under control by aggressive drug therapy, there will be ample time to reassess the clinical situation. In the unlikely event that the patient does indeed lose weight and continues to exercise and diet, step-down therapy can be considered.

Drug Therapy

Blockers of the Renin-Angiotensin-Aldosterone System (RAAS)

Blockers of RAAS, either ACE inhibitors or angiotensin receptor blockers (ARBs), have become a cornerstone in the management of the hypertensive diabetic patient. Both of these drug classes have been shown to favorably influence surrogate endpoints, such as reducing the occurrence of new-onset diabetes, to decrease microalbuminuria, to slow down progression from microproteinuria to macroproteinuria, and to slow down the decline in renal function. Outcome data in diabetic nephropathy are more solid for ACE inhibitors in type 1 diabetes and for ARBs in type 2 diabetes. The ADA guidelines initially, therefore, stated that ACE inhibitors were the drug of choice in patients with type 1 diabetes and ARBs in patients with type 2 diabetes. However, more recently the overall evidence has been deemed to be sufficient to motivate the ADA to change their statement, and to extend the indication of both of these drug classes for the whole spectrum of hypertensive/diabetic renal disease [101].

As discussed above, microalbuminuria is a marker for endothelial dysfunction and, as such, closely parallels not only target organ disease in the kidneys, but also elsewhere in the vascular tree, such as, the heart, the retina, and the brain. Blockade of RAAS either by an ACE inhibitor or by an ARB has been shown to be beneficial for the whole spectrum of hypertensive/diabetic heart disease, cerebrovascular disease as well as diabetic retinopathy. Given the unequivocal benefits of RAAS blockers in the diabetic hypertensive patient, one may ask whether any controversial or unresolved issues remain pertaining to these drugs.

Hyporeninemic Hypoaldosteronism. It is not uncommon for diabetic hypertensive patients to exhibit a feature called hyporeninemic hypoaldosteronism, i.e. inappropriately low activity of RAAS. These patients' blood pressure does not respond well to monotherapy with RAAS blockers, although ACE inhibitors or ARBs may still be vasculoprotective. Indeed, monotherapy with any drug class rarely gets blood pressure to goal in diabetic hypertensive patients; most often two or more drugs need to be combined.

Combination of RAAS Blockers. Should ARBs and ACE inhibitors be combined in a hypertensive patient with diabetic nephropathy? As a general rule, this combination has little if any additive effect on blood pressure, but may be synergistic with regard to reducing microproteinuria [102] and also, as was shown in the CHARM study [103], be beneficial in patients with congestive heart failure. As a rule, if blood pressure is at goal and the diabetic hypertensive patient still has significant microproteinuria, the combination of an ARB with an ACE inhibitor should be strongly considered if maximum doses of monotherapy of one drug have proven inefficacious.

Renal Impairment. Utmost caution is required in the diabetic hypertensive patient with renal impairment. An increase in creatinine and potassium are not an uncommon consequence of the RAAS blockade, occurring more commonly with ACE inhibitors than with ARBs. These adverse events can also be triggered by unforeseeable factors such as dehydration, concomitant drugs such as Cox 2 inhibitors, nonsteroidal anti-inflammatory drugs, i.v. contrast, etc. Also, as the disease and renal failure progress, a dose of an ACE inhibitor that was previously well tolerated may become inappropriate in a given patient. Of note, a small increase in creatinine (up to 20–25%) is acceptable after initiation of therapy with a blocker of the renin-angiotensin system and has even been deemed to be 'nephroprotective'. However, such therapy in diabetic patients at risk mandates a close monitoring of creatinine and electrolytes.

Aldosterone Antagonists. Aldosterone antagonists such as spironolactone and eplerenone can be exceedingly helpful in selected patients [104–109]. These drugs have been shown to reduce target organ disease and surrogate endpoints, such as microproteinuria and left ventricular hypertrophy [107]. Eplerenone has a cleaner adverse effect profile than does spironolactone in that it does not seem to cause gynecomastia and perhaps also is associated with less hyperkalemia [106]. However, since the diabetic hypertensive patient is prone to hyperkalemia (hyporeninemic hypoaldosteronism, renal impairment and/or ACE inhibitor/ARB treatment), these drugs should be used cautiously in low doses only and potassium and creatinine will have to be monitored frequently.

Calcium Antagonists

Calcium antagonists as a class are efficacious and dependable antihypertensive agents and have been shown to be at least as beneficial in diabetic hypertensive patients as is conventional therapy [110]. When used in monotherapy, non-dihydropyridine calcium antagonists such as verapamil and diltiazem have an edge over the dihydropyridines because they have been shown to decrease proteinuria almost to the same extent as the ACE inhibitors. In contrast, although proteinuria also decreases with the long-acting dihydropyridine, the renal benefits of these drugs are less well documented.

We did a meta-analysis of all available studies (n = 14) that reported outcome in diabetic hypertensive patients and used calcium antagonists [110]. Compared with conventional therapy, calcium antagonists had similar effects on coronary heart disease, but reduced the risk of stroke somewhat better (OR 0.87, 95% CI 0.74–1.2). Calcium antagonists, however, in this population showed a lesser reduction of the risk of congestive heart failure (OR 1.33). Similarly, when compared to blockers of the renin-angiotensin system, calcium antagonists were less effective in preventing heart failure (OR = 1.43), but had a similar beneficial effect on stroke, coronary heart disease and total mortality. Thus, calcium antagonists were safe and effective in reducing cardiovascular morbidity and mortality in diabetic hypertensive patients, although their use was associated with a lesser reduction of the risk of heart failure when compared to other treatment modalities.

Since a blocker of the RAAS is almost mandatory in the diabetic hypertensive patient, the question comes up whether as a second step a dihydropyridine calcium antagonist (such as amlodipine) or a non-dihydropyridine drug (such as verapamil) should be added. Very little data are available to look at this question. In one Italian study, proteinuria was reduced somewhat better by the verapamil/ACE inhibitor combination than by the amlodipine/ACE inhibitor combination, and there was also a qualitative difference in proteinuria favoring the non-dihydropyridine/ACE inhibitor combination [111].

Overall, calcium antagonists are extremely useful in the management of the diabetic hypertensive patient because of their consistency in lowering blood pressure regardless of co-morbidity, concomitant medication, salt intake, race, age, diet, activity of RAAS and their being metabolically neutral. In order to get blood pressure to goal, add-on therapy with a calcium antagonist is commonly needed.

Beta Blockers

As a general rule, beta blockers should not be used as first-line therapy in the diabetic hypertensive patient, although they are attractive as add on drugs in selected patients. Sympathetic activity is commonly enhanced in diabetes and coronary artery disease is often present, which are both favorably influenced by a beta- blocker. In the UKPDS study [96], the outcome was similar whether patients were randomized to a beta blocker or an ACE inhibitor. However, in this study the risk of coronary artery disease was not significantly reduced by either of the two drug classes.

The reason beta blockers are not considered ideal drugs for the diabetic hypertensive patient lies in their unfavorable effect on endocrine metabolic findings. Beta-blockers have been shown to increase triglycerides, lower HDL cholesterol, worsen insulin resistance, lead to a systemic weight gain and mask hypoglycemia. As a class, beta blockers have never been shown to reduce heart attacks or strokes in uncomplicated hypertension [112]. In the recent Anglo Scandinavian Cardiac Outcomes Trial (ASCOT), the amlodipine-based regimen was compared to the atenolol-based regimen in 19,257 hypertensive patients with at least one additional risk factor. The atenolol-based regimen prevented less cardiovascular events than the amlodipine-based regimen [113].

Beta blockers were not included in the recent NICE and AHA guidelines as an optional choice for the initial treatment of hypertension [20, 114]. This is clearly justified for elderly hypertensive patients, but not justified for young hypertensive patients [115]. The controversy regarding the role of beta blockers in hypertension still exists and the recent ESH/ECS guidelines left this group of drugs as one of the first-choice options [24]. It is noteworthy that not all beta blockers are created equal with regard to hemodynamic and endocrine metabolic findings. Carvedilol, an alpha-beta blocker has been shown to exert a more favorable effect on some of these parameters than do traditional beta blockers. Specifically, carvedilol when compared to metoprolol did improve insulin sensitivity as measured by glucose infusion rate, metabolic clearance rate, and insulin sensitivity index in nondiabetic patients, carvedilol also improved fasting glucose levels, glycosylated hemoglobin and insulin level in diabetic hypertensive patients [116]. These finding were recently corroborated by the GEMINI study [117], in which patients were prospectively randomized to either metoprolol or carvedilol, again showing a significant difference in glycemic control favoring carvedilol when compared to metoprolol. As a general rule, the use of beta blockers in diabetic patients should be restricted to patients who have indications for this drug class such as symptoms of sympathetic excess, tachycardia, coronary artery disease or as add-on therapy for uncontrolled hypertension. If a beta blocker is to be used in the diabetic hypertensive patient, carvedilol may be the drug of choice.

Diuretics

Thiazide diuretics have been, are and will be a cornerstone in the antihypertensive arsenal. Their efficacy has been documented in numerous outcome studies in uncomplicated hypertensive patients as well as in diabetic hypertensive patients. However, we do not think that they should be used indiscriminately in this patient population. Diuretics have been well documented to have negative effects on endocrine metabolic findings such as insulin resistance and electrolytes. The addition of an ACE inhibitor or possibly an ARB to a thiazide diuretic has been shown to mitigate the negative endocrine/metabolic effects to some extent [118]. However, in the INVEST study [119], the addition of a diuretic in a dose-dependent way increased the risk of new onset diabetes, and this was true whether the patient was on verapamil or atenolol.

As a general rule, thiazide diuretics are excellent antihypertensives but poor diuretics. In contrast, the loop diuretics are excellent diuretics but poor antihypertensives. Thus, although loop diuretics may have less diabetogenic effects than the thiazides, there is little reason for their use in diabetic patients, unless the increase in creatinine dictates so. Hyperuricemia and gout are common clinical complications in the diabetic patient. Thiazide diuretics further increase uric acid and their indiscriminant use may trigger a gout attack in a susceptible patient.

Diuretics have been documented to protect against strokes better than most other drug classes [120]. As such, they should be part of the cocktail in all patients with cerebrovascular disease or at high risk for cerebrovascular disease. Diuretic may also decrease renal protein excretion in diabetic hypertensive patients. In a recent study the thiazide-like diuretic indapamide was as effective as an ACE inhibitor in reducing urine albumin excretion [121]. The unfavorable effects of diuretics on glucose metabolism were not translated to increased cardiovascular morbidity and mortality during the follow-up of few years [122]. Recently, a long follow up (15 years) of the SHEP study showed that the diabetogenic effect of thiazide had no impact on cardiovascular morbidity and mortality [123]. As with most drug classes used in hypertension, the long-tem safety of diuretics remains uncertain. This means that in the diabetic hypertensive patient they should be used in low doses and in combination with other drugs such as ACE inhibitors and ARBs only.

Alpha Blockers

Alpha blockers have been shown to exert a favorable effect on metabolic endocrine parameters in that they improve insulin resistance, decrease total cholesterol, increase HDL, and decrease LDL cholesterol. Despite these seemingly favorable surrogate endpoint effects, the ALLHAT study has documented superiority of chlorthalidone in preventing coronary heart disease and congestive heart failure [124]. As a class, these drugs should no longer be used for initial therapy in uncomplicated hypertension. However, they may be useful agents as third and fourth step therapy and in patients with symptoms of prostatisin.

Combination Therapy

As discussed above, a RAAS blocker, either an ACE inhibitor or an ARB, represents the cornerstone of the antihypertensive arsenal in the diabetic hypertensive patient. As a second step, we think a calcium antagonist should be added, although some authorities (including the American Diabetes Association and the National Kidney Foundation) prefer a low dose of a thiazide diuretic as a second step. Regardless of this controversy, triple therapy (the 'holy trinity') in general will consist of a RAAS blocker, a calcium antagonist and a low dose of a thiazide diuretic. In monotherapy a non-dihydropyridine calcium antagonist should be preferred over the dihydropyridines. Once an ACE inhibitor is combined with a calcium antagonist, the difference between dihydropyridine and non-dihydropyridine is less pronounced although reduction of microproteins has been better documented with a verapamil/ACE inhibitor than with an amlodipine/ACE inhibitor combination. A beta blocker, preferentially carvedilol, can be used as a second step in patients with coronary artery disease or other indications for beta blockade. Carvedilol can also be added to the standard triple combination (blocker of the renin-angiotensin system, calcium antagonist, diuretic) if needed. Caution should be exerted in combining beta blockers with a non-dihydropyridines calcium antagonist because both of these drug classes cause bradycardia, may prolong the AV interval, and rarely trigger AV block.

Additional add-on therapies in patients on quadruple therapy are the alpha blockers and/or anti-adrenergic agents. We would like to emphasize, however, that combination therapy by and large is not evidence-based medicine. There are no outcome studies comparing one combination with the other in hypertension, not to speak of the diabetic hypertensive patient. Combination therapy, therefore, remains empirical and has to be based on clinical reasoning.

Adjunctive Therapy

Lipid-Lowering Agents

When event rates in diabetic cohort of randomized trials are scrutinized [125], it becomes increasingly clear that statins are efficacious in reducing events in this high-risk population. Simvastatin has been shown to reduce the rate of coronary heart disease by about 50% when compared to placebo in the diabetic cohort. In the recent CARDS study, 2,838 diabetic patients with a mean LDL at baseline of 118 mg/dl later were randomized atorvastatin or placebo [126]. After a median follow-up of about 4 years, there was a 37% reduction in the primary endpoint (acute coronary artery disease, death, non-fatal MI, unstable angina, cardiac arrest, coronary revascularization or stroke). Strokes were reduced by 48% and total mortality by 27%. The study was halted due to benefits of atorvastatin in patients with type 2 diabetes.

The recent guidelines of the American College of Physicians stated that lipid-lowering therapy should be used for primary prevention of macrovascular complications in all patients with type 2 diabetes and one or more cardiovascular risk factors, i.e. hypertension [127]. We wholeheartedly concur and recommend that all diabetic hypertensive patients receive statin therapy regardless of their lipid levels.

Antihypertensive Therapy and New-Onset Diabetes

Ever since the pioneering observation of Colin Dollery [128, 129] more than 20 years ago, a variety of studies documented that long-term diuretic therapy diminishes glucose tolerance and increases the risk of new onset diabetes. Conversely, as we learned from recent trials, treatment with antihypertensive drugs such as blockers of the renin-angiotensin system or calcium antagonists seem to decrease this risk [130, 131]. Compared to diuretics or 'conventional' (diuretic and/or beta blocker) therapy, blockers of the renin-angiotensin system, and to a lesser extent calcium antagonists, reduced the risk of new-onset diabetes substantially. The recent Antihypertensive Treatment and Lipid Profile in a North of Sweden Efficacy Evaluation (ALPINE) [132] study was designed to compare the effects of antihypertensive therapy on glucose metabolism in almost 400 patients with uncomplicated hypertension who had never been treated previously. Patients were randomized to either an ARB (with addition of calcium antagonist, if needed) or to a thiazide diuretic (and a beta blocker, if needed). After only 1 year of follow-up, 18 patients in the diuretic arm reached diagnostic criteria of the metabolic syndrome and 9 had developed frank diabetes. The corresponding numbers in the angiotensin receptor blocker arm were 5 and 1.

In the Antihypertensive and Lipid-Lowering Treatment to Prevent Heart Attack (ALLHAT) [133] study, about 10% of the total study population of patients developed new-onset diabetes during the 4–6 years' duration of the study. Of note, the risk of becoming diabetic was between 40 and 65% higher in patients on chlorthalidone-based therapy than in patients on lisinopril-based therapy, and between 18 and 30% higher in patients on chlorthalidone than in those on amlodipine.

Verdecchia et al. [134] report an up to 16-year follow-up of almost 800 initially untreated hypertensive patients, 6.5% of whom had diabetes at the onset, and 5.8% of whom developed new-onset diabetes throughout the study. The fasting blood sugar at entry as well as diuretic treatment on follow-up were independent, powerful predictors of new-onset diabetes ($p < 0.0001$ and $p < 0.004$, respectively). Most importantly, compared to subjects who never developed diabetes, the risk for cardiovascular disease during the follow-up was very similar in patients who developed diabetes (OR 2.92, 95% CI 1.33–6.41, $p = 0.007$) and in the group that had pre-existing diabetes (OR 3.57, 95% CI.1.65–7.73, $p = 0.001$). Patients with new-onset diabetes and those with a prior diagnosis of diabetes were almost three times as likely to develop subsequent cardiovascular disease than those who remained free of diabetes. These provocative findings not only show again that antihypertensive therapy with a thiazide diuretic confers a substantial risk of new onset diabetes, but more importantly that patients who have become diabetic will suffer all the adverse sequelae of this disease. Conceivably, the combination of a diuretic and an ACE inhibitor may confer a lesser risk of new onset diabetes. At least in a small short-term study ACE inhibitors seemed to prevent the metabolic deleterious effect of diuretic thiazide [118].

Of special interest in this context is the recently reported VALUE study in which a calcium antagonist strategy (amlodipine) was compared to an ARB strategy (valsartan) in more than 15,000 hypertensive patients [100]. New-onset diabetes, not a pre-specified endpoint, was 23% less common in the valsartan arm than in the amlodipine arm. Not surprisingly, drugs that block the renin-angiotensin system prevent hypokalemia and/or diminish the activity of the sympathetic nervous system are more favorable in terms of new-onset diabetes than drugs that are either metabolically neutral (calcium antagonists) or those that stimulate (diuretics) these physiologic systems. Indeed, hyperkalemia was almost twice as common in the amlodipine arm than in the valsartan arm.

Conclusion

The growing prevalence of diabetes and the metabolic syndrome underscores the need for therapies that reduce CVD risk factors while lowering plasma glucose. Hypoglycemic agents have disparate effects on the CVD risk factors.

References

1   Grossman E, Messerli FH: Diabetic and hypertensive heart disease. Ann Intern Med 1996;125: 304–310.
2   Gress TW, Nieto FJ, Shahar E, Wofford MR, Brancati FL: Hypertension and antihypertensive therapy as risk factors for type 2 diabetes mellitus. Atherosclerosis Risk in Communities Study. N Engl J Med 2000;342:905–912.
3   Stamler J, Vaccaro O, Neaton JD, Wentworth D: Diabetes, other risk factors, and 12-yr cardiovascular mortality for men screened in the Multiple Risk Factor Intervention Trial. Diabetes Care 1993;16:434–444.
4   Haffner SJ, Cassells H: Hyperglycemia as a cardiovascular risk factor. Am J Med 2003;115(suppl 8A): 6S–11S.
5   Brown MJ, Castaigne A, de Leeuw PW, et al: Influence of diabetes and type of hypertension on response to antihypertensive treatment. Hypertension 2000;35:1038–1042.
6   Messerli FH, Grossman E, Leonetti G: Antihypertensive therapy and new onset diabetes. J Hypertens 2004;22:1845–1847.
7   Harris MI, Flegal KM, Cowie CC, et al: Prevalence of diabetes, impaired fasting glucose, and impaired glucose tolerance in US adults. The Third National Health and Nutrition Examination Survey, 1988–1994. Diabetes Care 1998;21:518–524.
8   Drivsholm T, Ibsen H, Schroll M, Davidsen M, Borch-Johnsen K: Increasing prevalence of diabetes mellitus and impaired glucose tolerance among 60-year-old Danes. Diabet Med 2001;18: 126–132.

9   Pan XR, Yang WY, Li GW, Liu J: Prevalence of diabetes and its risk factors in China, 1994. National Diabetes Prevention and Control Cooperative Group. Diabetes Care 1997;20: 1664–1669.

10   Ramachandran A, Snehalatha C, Latha E, Vijay V, Viswanathan M: Rising prevalence of NIDDM in an urban population in India. Diabetologia 1997;40:232–237.

11   King H, Aubert RE, Herman WH: Global burden of diabetes, 1995–2025: prevalence, numerical estimates, and projections. Diabetes Care 1998;21:1414–1431.

12   Zimmet P, Alberti KG, Shaw J: Global and societal implications of the diabetes epidemic. Nature 2001;414:782–787.

13   Harris SB, Gittelsohn J, Hanley A, et al: The prevalence of NIDDM and associated risk factors in native Canadians. Diabetes Care 1997;20:185–187.

14   Report of the Expert Committee on the Diagnosis and Classification of Diabetes Mellitus. Diabetes Care 1997;20:1183–1197.

15   Dunstan DW, Zimmet PZ, Welborn TA, et al: The rising prevalence of diabetes and impaired glucose tolerance: the Australian Diabetes, Obesity and Lifestyle Study. Diabetes Care 2002;25: 829–834.

16   Isomaa B, Almgren P, Tuomi T, et al: Cardiovascular morbidity and mortality associated with the metabolic syndrome. Diabetes Care 2001;24:683–689.

17   Kearney PM, Whelton M, Reynolds K, Muntner P, Whelton PK, He J: Global burden of hypertension: analysis of worldwide data. Lancet 2005;365:217–223.

18   Sowers JR: Recommendations for special populations: diabetes mellitus and the metabolic syndrome. Am J Hypertens 2003;16:41S–45S.

19   Arauz-Pacheco C, Parrott MA, Raskin P: The treatment of hypertension in adult patients with diabetes. Diabetes Care 2002;25:134–147.

20   Rosendorff C, Black HR, Cannon CP, et al: Treatment of hypertension in the prevention and management of ischemic heart disease: a scientific statement from the American Heart Association Council for High Blood Pressure Research and the Councils on Clinical Cardiology and Epidemiology and Prevention. Circulation 2007;115:2761–2788.

21   Grossman E, Messerli FH, Goldbourt U: High blood pressure and diabetes mellitus: are all antihypertensive drugs created equal? Arch Intern Med 2000;160:2447–2452.

22   Shaw JE, Zimmet PZ, Hodge AM, et al: Impaired fasting glucose: how low should it go? Diabetes Care 2000;231:34–39.

23   Hu G, Qiao Q, Tuomilehto J, Balkau B, Borch-Johnsen K, Pyorala K: Prevalence of the metabolic syndrome and its relation to all-cause and cardiovascular mortality in nondiabetic European men and women. Arch Intern Med 2004;164:1066–1076.

24   Mancia G, De Backer G, Dominiczak A, et al: 2007 Guidelines for the Management of Arterial Hypertension: The Task Force for the Management of Arterial Hypertension of the European Society of Hypertension (ESH) and of the European Society of Cardiology (ESC). J Hypertens 2007;25:1105–1187.

25   Schillaci G, Pirro M, Vaudo G, et al: Prognostic value of the metabolic syndrome in essential hypertension. J Am Coll Cardiol 2004;43:1817–1822.

26   Sowers JR, Epstein M, Frohlich ED: Diabetes, hypertension, and cardiovascular disease: an update. Hypertension 2001;37:1053–1059.

27   Carrozza JP Jr, Kuntz RE, Fishman RF, Baim DS: Restenosis after arterial injury caused by coronary stenting in patients with diabetes mellitus. Ann Intern Med 1993;118:344–349.

28   Comparison of coronary bypass surgery with angioplasty in patients with multivessel disease. The Bypass Angioplasty Revascularization Investigation (BARI) Investigators. N Engl J Med 1996;335:217–225.

29   Nesto RW, Phillips RT, Kett KG, et al: Angina and exertional myocardial ischemia in diabetic and nondiabetic patients: assessment by exercise thallium scintigraphy. Ann Intern Med 1988;108: 170–175.

30   Haffner SM, Lehto S, Ronnemaa T, Pyörälä K, Laakso M: Mortality from coronary heart disease in subjects with type 2 diabetes and in nondiabetic subjects with and without prior myocardial infarction. N Engl J Med 1998;339:229–234.

31   Hoffman JI: A critical view of coronary reserve. Circulation 1987;75:I6–I11.

---

32 Grossman E, Rosenthal T: Hypertensive heart disease and the diabetic patient. Curr Opin Cardiol 1995;10:458–465.

33 Kannel WB, Dannenberg AL, Abbott RD: Unrecognized myocardial infarction and hypertension: the Framingham Study. Am Heart J 1985;109:581–585.

34 Assmann G, Schulte H: The Prospective Cardiovascular Munster (PROCAM) study: prevalence of hyperlipidemia in persons with hypertension and/or diabetes mellitus and the relationship to coronary heart disease. Am Heart J 1988;116:1713–1724.

35 Melina D, Colivicchi F, Melina G, Pristipino C: Prevalence of silent ST segment depression during long-term ambulatory electrocardiographic monitoring in asymptomatic diabetic patients with essential hypertension. Minerva Med 1993;84:301–305.

36 Kannel WB, Hjortland M, Castelli WP: Role of diabetes in congestive heart failure: the Framingham study. Am J Cardiol 1974;34:29–34.

37 Schannwell CM, Schneppenheim M, Perings S, Plehn G, Strauer BE: Left ventricular diastolic dysfunction as an early manifestation of diabetic cardiomyopathy. Cardiology 2002;98: 33–39.

38 Shapiro LM: Echocardiographic features of impaired ventricular function in diabetes mellitus. Br Heart J 1982;47:439–444.

39 Borow KM, Jaspan JB, Williams KA, Neumann A, Wolinski-Walley P, Lang RM: Myocardial mechanics in young adult patients with diabetes mellitus: effects of altered load, inotropic state and dynamic exercise. J Am Coll Cardiol 1990;15:1508–1517.

40 Mustonen JN, Uusitupa MI, Laakso M, et al: Left ventricular systolic function in middle-aged patients with diabetes mellitus. Am J Cardiol 1994;73:1202–1208.

41 Iwasaka T, Sugiura T, Abe Y, et al: Residual left ventricular pump function following acute myocardial infarction in postmenopausal diabetic women. Coron Artery Dis 1994;5:237–242.

42 Gustafsson I, Hildebrandt P: Early failure of the diabetic heart. Diabetes Care 2001;24:3–4.

43 Intensive blood-glucose control with sulphonylureas or insulin compared with conventional treatment and risk of complications in patients with type 2 diabetes (UKPDS 33). UK Prospective Diabetes Study (UKPDS) Group. Lancet 1998;352:837–853.

44 Shindler DM, Kostis JB, Yusuf S, et al: Diabetes mellitus, a predictor of morbidity and mortality in the Studies of Left Ventricular Dysfunction (SOLVD) trials and registry. Am J Cardiol 1996;77:1017–1020.

45 Blendea MC, McFarlane SI, Isenovic ER, Gick G, Sowers JR: Heart disease in diabetic patients. Curr Diab Rep 2003;3:223–229.

46 Malmberg K, Ryden L, Efendic S, et al: Randomized trial of insulin-glucose infusion followed by subcutaneous insulin treatment in diabetic patients with acute myocardial infarction (DIGAMI study): effects on mortality at 1 year. J Am Coll Cardiol 1995;26:57–65.

47 Henry P, Thomas F, Benetos A, Guize L: Impaired fasting glucose, blood pressure and cardiovascular disease mortality. Hypertension 2002;40:458–463.

48 Marroquin OC, Kip KE, Kelley DE, et al: Metabolic syndrome modifies the cardiovascular risk associated with angiographic coronary artery disease in women: a report from the Women's Ischemia Syndrome Evaluation. Circulation 2004;109:714–721.

49 Drayer JI, Gardin JM, Brewer DD, Weber MA: Disparate relationships between blood pressure and left ventricular mass in patients with and without left ventricular hypertrophy. Hypertension 1987;9:II61–II64.

50 Frohlich ED, Apstein C, Chobanian AV, et al: The heart in hypertension. N Engl J Med 1992;327:998–1008.

51 Mercadier JJ, Lompre AM, Wisnewsky C, et al: Myosin isoenzyme changes in several models of rat cardiac hypertrophy. Circ Res 1981;49:525–532.

52 Grossman E, Oren S, Messerli FH: Left ventricular mass and cardiac function in patients with essential hypertension. J Hum Hypertens 1994;8:417–421.

53 Devereux RB: Left ventricular diastolic dysfunction: early diastolic relaxation and late diastolic compliance. J Am Coll Cardiol 1989;13:337–339.

54 Gerdts E, Bjornstad H, Toft S, Devereux RB, Omvik P: Impact of diastolic Doppler indices on exercise capacity in hypertensive patients with electrocardiographic left ventricular hypertrophy (a LIFE substudy). J Hypertens 2002;20:1223–1229.

55   Grossman E, Oren S, Messerli FH: Left ventricular filling and stress response pattern in essential hypertension. Am J Med 1991;91:502–506.

56   Skaluba SJ, Litwin SE: Mechanisms of exercise intolerance: insights from tissue Doppler imaging. Circulation 2004;109:972–977.

57   Kannel WB, Castelli WP, McNamara PM, McKee PA, Feinleib M: Role of blood pressure in the development of congestive heart failure. The Framingham study. N Engl J Med 1972;287: 781–787.

58   Garty M, Shotan A, Gottlieb S, et al: The management, early and one year outcome in hospitalized patients with heart failure: a national Heart Failure Survey in Israel–HFSIS 2003. Isr Med Assoc J 2007;9:227–233.

59   Lewis BS, Shotan A, Gottlieb S, et al: Late mortality and determinants in patients with heart failure and preserved systolic left ventricular function: the Israel Nationwide Heart Failure Survey. Isr Med Assoc J 2007;9:234–238.

60   Haider AW, Larson MG, Franklin SS, Levy D: Systolic blood pressure, diastolic blood pressure, and pulse pressure as predictors of risk for congestive heart failure in the Framingham Heart Study. Ann Intern Med 2003;138:10–16.

61   Kannel WB: Prevalence and natural history of electrocardiographic left ventricular hypertrophy. Am J Med 1983;75:4–11.

62   van Hoeven KH, Factor SM: A comparison of the pathological spectrum of hypertensive, diabetic, and hypertensive-diabetic heart disease. Circulation 1990;82:848–855.

63   Grossman E, Shemesh J, Shamiss A, Thaler M, Carroll J, Rosenthal T: Left ventricular mass in diabetes-hypertension. Arch Intern Med 1992;152:1001–1004.

64   Venco A, Grandi A, Barzizza F, Finardi G: Echocardiographic features of hypertensive-diabetic heart muscle disease. Cardiology 1987;74:28–34.

65   Sahai A, Ganguly PK: Congestive heart failure in diabetes with hypertension may be due to uncoupling of the atrial natriuretic peptide receptor-effector system in the kidney basolateral membrane. Am Heart J 1991;122:164–170.

66   Lea JP, Nicholas SB: Diabetes mellitus and hypertension: key risk factors for kidney disease. J Natl Med Assoc 2002;94(8 suppl):7S–15S.

67   Chaiken RL, Eckert-Norton M, Bard M, et al: Hyperfiltration in African-American patients with type 2 diabetes: cross-sectional and longitudinal data. Diabetes Care 1998;21:2129–2134.

68   Burnier M, Zanchi A: Blockade of the renin-angiotensin-aldosterone system: a key therapeutic strategy to reduce renal and cardiovascular events in patients with diabetes. J Hypertens 2006;24: 11–25.

69   Gerstein HC, Mann JF, Yi Q, et al: Albuminuria and risk of cardiovascular events, death, and heart failure in diabetic and nondiabetic individuals. JAMA 2001;286:421–426.

70   National High Blood Pressure Education Program Working Group report on hypertension and chronic renal failure. Arch Intern Med 1991;151:1280–1287.

71   Klag MJ, Whelton PK, Randall BL, et al: Blood pressure and end-stage renal disease in men. N Engl J Med 1996;334:13–18.

72   Bakris GL, Williams M, Dworkin L, et al: Preserving renal function in adults with hypertension and diabetes: a consensus approach. National Kidney Foundation Hypertension and Diabetes Executive Committees Working Group. Am J Kidney Dis 2000;36:646–661.

73   Beckman JA, Creager MA, Libby P: Diabetes and atherosclerosis: epidemiology, pathophysiology, and management. JAMA 2002;287:2570–2581.

74   Newman AB, Siscovick DS, Manolio TA, et al: Ankle-arm index as a marker of atherosclerosis in the Cardiovascular Health Study. Cardiovascular Heart Study (CHS) Collaborative Research Group. Circulation 1993;88:837–845.

75   Abbott RD, Brand FN, Kannel WB: Epidemiology of some peripheral arterial findings in diabetic men and women: experiences from the Framingham Study. Am J Med 1990;88:376–381.

76   Hiatt WR, Hirsch AT, Regensteiner JG, Brass EP: Clinical trials for claudication: assessment of exercise performance, functional status, and clinical end points. Vascular clinical trialists. Circulation 1995;92:614–621.

77   Meijer WT, Hoes AW, Rutgers D, Bots ML, Hofman A, Grobbee DE: Peripheral arterial disease in the elderly: The Rotterdam Study. Arterioscler Thromb Vasc Biol 1998;18:185–192.

78   Kallio M, Forsblom C, Groop PH, Groop L, Lepantalo M: Development of new peripheral arterial occlusive disease in patients with type 2 diabetes during a mean follow-up of 11 years. Diabetes Care 2003;26:1241–1245.

79   Jude EB, Oyibo SO, Chalmers N, Boulton AJ: Peripheral arterial disease in diabetic and nondiabetic patients: a comparison of severity and outcome. Diabetes Care 2001;24:1433–1437.

80   Beks PJ, Mackaay AJ, de Neeling JN, de Vries H, Bouter LM, Heine RJ: Peripheral arterial disease in relation to glycaemic level in an elderly Caucasian population: the Hoorn study. Diabetologia 1995;38:86–96.

81   Uusitupa MI, Niskanen LK, Siitonen O, Voutilainen E, Pyorala K: 5-year incidence of atherosclerotic vascular disease in relation to general risk factors, insulin level, and abnormalities in lipoprotein composition in non-insulin-dependent diabetic and nondiabetic subjects. Circulation 1990;82:27–36.

82   Hooi JD, Kester AD, Stoffers HE, Overdijk MM, van Ree JW, Knottnerus JA: Incidence of and risk factors for asymptomatic peripheral arterial occlusive disease: a longitudinal study. Am J Epidemiol 2001;153:666–672.

83   Dormandy JA, Rutherford RB: Management of peripheral arterial disease (PAD). TASC Working Group: TransAtlantic Inter-Society Concensus (TASC). J Vasc Surg 2000;31:S1–S296.

84   Friedlander AH, Maeder LA: The prevalence of calcified carotid artery atheromas on the panoramic radiographs of patients with type 2 diabetes mellitus. Oral Surg Oral Med Oral Pathol Oral Radiol Endod 2000;89:420–424.

85   Himmelmann A, Hansson L, Svensson A, Harmsen P, Holmgren C, Svanborg A: Predictors of stroke in the elderly. Acta Med Scand 1988;224:439–443.

86   Tanne D, Goldbourt U, Koton S, et al: A national survey of acute cerebrovascular disease in Israel: burden, management, outcome and adherence to guidelines. Isr Med Assoc J 2006;8:3–7.

87   Folsom AR, Rasmussen ML, Chambless LE, et al: Prospective associations of fasting insulin, body fat distribution, and diabetes with risk of ischemic stroke. The Atherosclerosis Risk in Communities (ARIC) Study Investigators. Diabetes Care 1999;22:1077–1083.

88   Jamrozik K, Broadhurst RJ, Forbes S, Hankey GJ, Anderson CS: Predictors of death and vascular events in the elderly: the Perth Community Stroke Study. Stroke 2000;31:863–868.

89   Jorgensen H, Nakayama H, Raaschou HO, Olsen TS: Stroke in patients with diabetes. The Copenhagen Stroke Study. Stroke 1994;25:1977–1984.

90   You RX, McNeil JJ, O'Malley HM, Davis SM, Thrift AG, Donnan GA: Risk factors for stroke due to cerebral infarction in young adults. Stroke 1997;28:1913–1918.

91   Luchsinger JA, Tang MX, Stern Y, Shea S, Mayeux R: Diabetes mellitus and risk of Alzheimer's disease and dementia with stroke in a multiethnic cohort. Am J Epidemiol 2001;154:635–641.

92   Hankey GJ, Jamrozik K, Broadhurst RJ, et al: Long-term risk of first recurrent stroke in the Perth Community Stroke Study. Stroke 1998;29:2491–2500.

93   Tuomilehto J, Rastenyte D, Jousilahti P, Sarti C, Vartiainen E: Diabetes mellitus as a risk factor for death from stroke: prospective study of the middle-aged Finnish population. Stroke 1996;27: 210–215.

94   Lewington S, Clarke R, Qizilbash N, Peto R, Collins R: Age-specific relevance of usual blood pressure to vascular mortality: a meta-analysis of individual data for one million adults in 61 prospective studies. Lancet 2002;360:1903–1913.

95   Staessen JA, Gasowski J, Wang JG, et al: Risks of untreated and treated isolated systolic hypertension in the elderly: meta-analysis of outcome trials. Lancet 2000;355:865–872.

96   UK Prospective Diabetes Study Group: Tight blood pressure control and risk of macrovascular and microvascular complications in type 2 diabetes: UKPDS 38. BMJ 1998;317:703–713.

97   Knowler WC, Bennett PH, Ballintine EJ: Increased incidence of retinopathy in diabetics with elevated blood pressure: a six-year follow-up study in Pima Indians. N Engl J Med 1980;302: 645–650.

98   Messerli FH, Mancia G, Conti CR, et al: Dogma disputed: can aggressively lowering blood pressure in hypertensive patients with coronary artery disease be dangerous? Ann Intern Med 2006;144:884–893.

99   Sjostrom L, Lindroos AK, Peltonen M, et al: Lifestyle, diabetes, and cardiovascular risk factors 10 years after bariatric surgery. N Engl J Med 2004;351:2683–2693.

100   Julius S, Kjeldsen SE, Weber M, et al: Outcomes in hypertensive patients at high cardiovascular risk treated with regimens based on valsartan or amlodipine: the VALUE randomised trial. Lancet 2004;363:2022–2031.
101   Standards of medical care in diabetes. Diabetes Care 2004;27(suppl 1):S15–S35.
102   Rossing K, Jacobsen P, Pietraszek L, Parving HH: Renoprotective effects of adding angiotensin II receptor blocker to maximal recommended doses of ACE inhibitor in diabetic nephropathy: a randomized double-blind crossover trial. Diabetes Care 2003;26:2268–2274.
103   Granger CB, McMurray JJ, Yusuf S, et al: Effects of candesartan in patients with chronic heart failure and reduced left-ventricular systolic function intolerant to angiotensin-converting-enzyme inhibitors: the CHARM-Alternative trial. Lancet 2003;362:772–776.
104   Calhoun DA: Low-dose aldosterone blockade as a new treatment paradigm for controlling resistant hypertension. J Clin Hypertens (Greenwich) 2007;9(suppl 1):19–24.
105   Chapman N, Dobson J, Wilson S, et al: Effect of spironolactone on blood pressure in subjects with resistant hypertension. Hypertension 2007;49:839–845.
106   Croom KF, Perry CM: Eplerenone: a review of its use in essential hypertension. Am J Cardiovasc Drugs 2005;5:51–69.
107   Epstein M: Adding spironolactone to conventional antihypertensives reduces albuminuria in patients with diabetic nephropathy. Nat Clin Pract Nephrol 2006;2:310–311.
108   Goodfriend TL: Treating resistant hypertension with a neglected old drug. Hypertension 2007;49:763–764.
109   Sharabi Y, Adler E, Shamis A, Nussinovitch N, Markovitz A, Grossman E: Efficacy of add-on aldosterone receptor blocker in uncontrolled hypertension. Am J Hypertens 2006;19:750–755.
110   Grossman E, Messerli FH: Are calcium antagonists beneficial in diabetic patients with hypertension? Am J Med 2004;116:44–49.
111   Boero R, Rollino C, Massara C, et al: The verapamil versus amlodipine in nondiabetic nephropathies treated with trandolapril (VVANNTT) study. Am J Kidney Dis 2003;42:67–75.
112   Messerli FH, Grossman E, Goldbourt U: Are beta-blockers efficacious as first-line therapy for hypertension in the elderly? A systematic review. JAMA 1998;279:1903–1907.
113   Dahlof B, Sever PS, Poulter NR, et al: Prevention of cardiovascular events with an antihypertensive regimen of amlodipine adding perindopril as required versus atenolol adding bendroflumethiazide as required in the Anglo-Scandinavian Cardiac Outcomes Trial-Blood Pressure Lowering Arm (ASCOT-BPLA): a multicentre randomised controlled trial. Lancet 2005;366:895–906.
114   Sever P: New hypertension guidelines from the National Institute for Health and Clinical Excellence and the British Hypertension Society. J Renin Angiotensin Aldosterone Syst 2006;7:61–63.
115   Khan N, McAlister FA: Re-examining the efficacy of beta-blockers for the treatment of hypertension: a meta-analysis. CMAJ 2006;174:1737–1742.
116   Giugliano D, Acampora R, Marfella R, et al: Metabolic and cardiovascular effects of carvedilol and atenolol in non-insulin-dependent diabetes mellitus and hypertension: a randomized, controlled trial. Ann Intern Med 1997;126:955–959.
117   Bakris GL, Fonseca V, Katholi RE, et al: Metabolic effects of carvedilol vs. metoprolol in patients with type 2 diabetes mellitus and hypertension: a randomized controlled trial. JAMA 2004;292: 2227–2236.
118   Shamiss A, Carroll J, Peleg E, Grossman E, Rosenthal T: The effect of enalapril with and without hydrochlorothiazide on insulin sensitivity and other metabolic abnormalities of hypertensive patients with NIDDM. Am J Hypertens 1995;8:276–281.
119   Cooper-Dehoff R, Cohen JD, Bakris GL, et al: Predictors of development of diabetes mellitus in patients with coronary artery disease taking antihypertensive medications (findings from the INternational VErapamil SR-Trandolapril STudy [INVEST]). Am J Cardiol 2006;98:890–894.
120   Messerli FH, Grossman E, Lever AF: Do thiazide diuretics confer specific protection against strokes? Arch Intern Med 2003;163:2557–2560.
121   Puig JG, Marre M, Kokot F, et al: Efficacy of indapamide SR compared with enalapril in elderly hypertensive patients with type 2 diabetes. Am J Hypertens 2007;20:90–97.
122   Barzilay JI, Davis BR, Cutler JA, et al: Fasting glucose levels and incident diabetes mellitus in older nondiabetic adults randomized to receive 3 different classes of antihypertensive treatment:

a report from the Antihypertensive and Lipid-Lowering Treatment to Prevent Heart Attack Trial (ALLHAT). Arch Intern Med 2006;166:2191–2201.

123   Kostis JB, Wilson AC, Freudenberger RS, Cosgrove NM, Pressel SL, Davis BR: Long-term effect of diuretic-based therapy on fatal outcomes in subjects with isolated systolic hypertension with and without diabetes. Am J Cardiol 2005;95:29–35.

124   Messerli FH: Implications of discontinuation of doxazosin arm of ALLHAT: Antihypertensive and Lipid-Lowering Treatment to Prevent Heart Attack Trial. Lancet 2000;355:863–864.

125   Sowers JR, Haffner S: Treatment of cardiovascular and renal risk factors in the diabetic hypertensive. Hypertension 2002;40:781–788.

126   Colhoun HM, Betteridge DJ, Durrington PN, et al: Rapid emergence of effect of atorvastatin on cardiovascular outcomes in the Collaborative Atorvastatin Diabetes Study (CARDS). Diabetologia 2005;48:2482–2485.

127   Snow V, Aronson MD, Hornbake ER, Mottur-Pilson C, Weiss KB: Lipid control in the management of type 2 diabetes mellitus: a clinical practice guideline from the American College of Physicians. Ann Intern Med 2004;140:644–649.

128   Lewis PJ, Kohner EM, Petrie A, Dollery CT: Deterioration of glucose tolerance in hypertensive patients on prolonged diuretic treatment. Lancet 1976;i:564–566.

129   Murphy MB, Lewis PJ, Kohner E, Schumer B, Dollery CT: Glucose intolerance in hypertensive patients treated with diuretics: a fourteen-year follow-up. Lancet 1982;2:1293–1295.

130   Mancia G, Grassi G, Zanchetti A: New-onset diabetes and antihypertensive drugs. J Hypertens 2006;24:3–10.

131   Yusuf S, Gerstein H, Hoogwerf B, et al: Ramipril and the development of diabetes. JAMA 2001;286:1882–1885.

132   Lindholm LH, Persson M, Alaupovic P, Carlberg B, Svensson A, Samuelsson O: Metabolic outcome during 1 year in newly detected hypertensives: results of the Antihypertensive Treatment and Lipid Profile in a North of Sweden Efficacy Evaluation (ALPINE study). J Hypertens 2003;21: 1563–1574.

133   Major outcomes in high-risk hypertensive patients randomized to angiotensin-converting enzyme inhibitor or calcium channel blocker vs. diuretic: The Antihypertensive and Lipid-Lowering Treatment to Prevent Heart Attack Trial (ALLHAT). JAMA 2002;288:2981–2997.

134   Verdecchia P, Reboldi G, Angeli F, et al: Adverse prognostic significance of new diabetes in treated hypertensive subjects. Hypertension 2004;43:963–969.

Prof. Ehud Grossman, MD
Internal Medicine D and Hypertension Unit, The Chaim Sheba Medical Center
Tel-Hashomer 52621 (Israel)
Tel. +972 3 530 2834, Fax +972 3 530 2835, E-Mail grosse@post.tau.ac.il

Fisman EZ, Tenenbaum A (eds): Cardiovascular Diabetology: Clinical, Metabolic and
Inflammatory Facets. Adv Cardiol. Basel, Karger, 2008, vol 45, pp 107–113

....

Impaired Glucose Metabolism and Cerebrovascular Diseases

David Tanne

Stroke Center, Department of Neurology Sheba Medical Center, Tel-Hashomer, and
Division of Epidemiology and Preventive Medicine, Sackler Faculty of Medicine,
Tel-Aviv University, Tel-Aviv, Israel

Abstract

Ischemic stroke and vascular cognitive impairment are leading causes of long-term disability and constitute a major public health burden and a significant economic burden to
health systems. An increasing body of evidence demonstrates that disorders of glucose
metabolism including diabetes, and the intermediate states of impaired fasting glucose and
impaired glucose tolerance, as well as the cluster of risk factors known as the metabolic syndrome, are important risk factors for ischemic stroke. The associations with accelerated cognitive decline and dementia are also discussed. Underlying pathogenetic mechanisms are
myriad but include insulin resistance, endothelial dysfunction, dyslipidemia, chronic inflammation, procoagulability, and impaired fibrinolysis. The high risk associated with diabetes
and other disorders of glucose metabolism carries important implications for preventive
strategies for cerebrovascular disease and vascular cognitive impairment that are currently
under investigation.

Stroke is a leading cause of long-term disability, a major public health burden, and a significant economic burden to health systems [1]. It constitutes the
second commonest cause of mortality worldwide and the third commonest
cause of mortality in more developed countries. The World Health Organization
estimates that about 15 million strokes occur annually worldwide and about
5 million deaths per year are due to stroke. Based on a recent population-based
study of all acute vascular events conducted in Oxford (The Oxford Vascular
Study), the relative incidence of cerebrovascular events is higher than that of
coronary events: the ratio is 1.2-fold higher overall and 1.4-fold higher for nonfatal strokes vs. coronary events [2].

Diabetes mellitus constitutes one of the major risk factors for stroke. Patients with type 2 diabetes are at increased risk of stroke with an increased relative risk ranging from 2- to 6-fold, and worsening glycemic control relates to stroke risk [3–10]. Diabetes particularly affects the risk of stroke among younger patients [11, 12]. In the stroke population younger than 55 years, diabetes increases the risk of stroke more than 10-fold [12]. Diabetes adversely affects cerebrovascular arterial circulation. Patients with diabetes have accelerated progression of carotid intima-media thickness, more extra- and intracranial atherosclerosis, and are prone to small vessel occlusive disease, affecting small penetrating arteries in the brain, and cardiac disease predisposing to embolic stroke. They are at increased risk, therefore, for all subtypes of ischemic stroke. They are also at increased cerebrovascular risk due to the effects of hyperglycemia on vascular tissues and coagulation, and aberrations in blood pressure regulation, lipid metabolism, endothelial function, vascular inflammation, lipid metabolism, smooth muscle cell proliferation, and fibrinolysis. Diabetes affects stroke outcome as well. It increases the risk of stroke-related dementia more than 3-fold [13], doubles the risk of recurrence [14], and increases total and stroke-related mortality [3].

Not only patients with diabetes are at increased risk of stroke but also patients with impaired fasting glucose or impaired glucose tolerance [15–19]. Among a cohort of about 14,000 patients with chronic coronary heart disease, we have found a J-shaped association between fasting plasma glucose and incident ischemic cerebrovascular events (fig. 1) [15]. As compared to those with fasting glucose 90–99 mg/dl, stroke incidence rates increased for levels 100–109 (adjusted OR 1.3) and 110–125 mg/dl (adjusted OR 1.6), with rising OR associated with increasing fasting glucose levels. Also patients with low fasting glucose levels (<80 mg/dl) exhibited a 1.5-fold increased risk of stroke, although the mechanisms underlying this association need yet to be elucidated. Similarly, among over 3,000 patients with a transient ischemic attack (TIA) or minor ischemic stroke that participated in the Dutch TIA Trial, stroke risk was nearly doubled in patients with impaired glucose tolerance compared with those with normal glucose levels and nearly tripled in diabetic patients [16]. Patients with low glucose levels also exhibited a 50% increased stroke risk.

Few studies, though not all, have suggested that insulin resistance may be associated with risk for stroke [17]. Emerging evidence has linked insulin resistance to the pathophysiologic derangements in type 2 diabetes mellitus that accelerates atherosclerosis. Analyses from the Third National Health and Nutrition Survey revealed that impaired insulin sensitivity assessed using the homeostasis model is independently associated with stroke, even after adjustment for glycemic control [18]. Among patients with recent stroke, 70% will have known diabetes, occult diabetes (detectable on an oral glucose tolerance

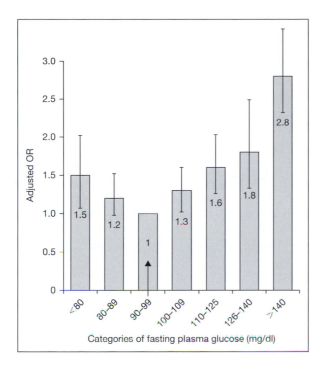

Fig. 1. Adjusted odds ratios (95% CI) for ischemic cerebrovascular disease by categories of fasting plasma glucose levels. Odds ratio for the 90–99 mg/dl category is defined as 1 (arrow). Modified from Tanne et al. [15].

test), or prediabetes [19]. Treatment of insulin resistance with weight loss, exercise, or medications can correct these derangements, and represent a promising approach to stroke prevention. Thiazolidinediones activate the peroxisome proliferator activated receptor-gamma (PPAR-γ) that functions as a transcription factor and modulates several genes involved in glucose and lipid metabolism, inflammation, cytokine production, and cell proliferation. A pilot study has found that the thiazolidinedione pioglitazone is effective for improving insulin sensitivity among patients with recent TIA or stroke and impaired insulin sensitivity [20], and an ongoing pivotal randomized clinical trial (Insulin Resistance Intervention after Stroke; IRIS trial) is currently assessing the efficacy of pioglitazone compared with placebo, for prevention of recurrent stroke and myocardial infarction among nondiabetic men and women with a recent ischemic stroke or TIA and insulin resistance.

Subjects with metabolic syndrome are at increased risk not only for ischemic heart disease but also for ischemic stroke [21–25]. In a prospective cohort of patients with chronic coronary heart disease, we have found that more than half the patients have metabolic syndrome or diabetes [21]. A significant increase in the risk of ischemic stroke or TIA was found in the presence of metabolic syndrome, even without diabetes. The presence of metabolic syndrome per se was associated with a 1.5-fold higher risk vs. a more than 2-fold higher risk associated with the presence of diabetes. Although both men and women with metabolic syndrome were at increased risk of ischemic stroke, relative odds were more pronounced in women then in men. The risk of ischemic stroke or TIA increased in an incremental fashion with an increasing number of components of the syndrome. The age- and sex-adjusted odds ratio for ischemic stroke or TIA among patients without diabetes was 2-fold greater in patients with 3 components of the metabolic syndrome present and as high as 5-fold greater in patients with all 5 components of metabolic syndrome present compared to patients without any of the components. Among patients from the same cohort, low high-density lipoprotein and high triglycerides [26] as well as inflammatory biomarkers such as C-reactive protein (CRP) and intracellular molecule-1 levels were found to be associated with an increased hazard for ischemic stroke [27, 28]. In a cohort of male civil servants and municipal employees free of cardiovascular disease and diabetes, low high-density lipoprotein concentrations and indices of body fat distribution predicted long-term stroke mortality, independent of the main mediators of the effect of obesity on health [9, 29, 30].

An increased risk of stroke among subjects with metabolic syndrome was observed in several other cohorts. A prospective study of subjects with hypertension without cardiovascular diseases found that metabolic syndrome was an independent predictor for both cardiovascular and cerebrovascular disease [24]. In a population-based cohort study with an average follow-up of 14 years from eastern Finland, the risk of any stroke was increased in men with metabolic syndrome in the absence of stroke, diabetes and cardiovascular disease at baseline [22]. Over 14 years of follow-up among subjects included in the Framingham Offspring Study, the relative risk of stroke in subjects with metabolic syndrome alone was 2.1, diabetes alone 2.5, and both 3.3 [31]. The population-attributable risk, owing to its greater prevalence, was greater for metabolic syndrome alone than for diabetes alone (19 vs. 7%), particularly in women (27 vs. 5%). In a study among middle-aged Japanese men and women, metabolic syndrome increased the risk of ischemic stroke 1.5-fold [25].

Impaired glucose metabolism is associated not only with stroke but also with changes in cognition. In type 2 diabetes cognitive changes mainly affect learning and memory, mental flexibility, and mental speed. Several large longitudinal population-based studies have shown that the rate of cognitive decline is accelerated in elderly people with type 2 diabetes. The determinants of this accelerated cognitive decline, however, are less clear. In a systematic review the incidence of any dementia was higher in those with diabetes than in those without [32]. The high-risk types included both Alzheimer's disease and vascular dementia. Among participants in the Israeli Ischemic Heart Disease study, diabetes in midlife was linked to dementia more than three decades later in the very old survivors of this large male cohort [33]. The findings of mechanistic studies suggest that vascular disease and alterations in glucose, insulin, and amyloid metabolism underlie the pathophysiology, but which of these mechanisms are clinically relevant is yet unclear. Both diabetes and insulin resistance per se were found to be associated with worse executive dysfunction in older persons [34, 35], and metabolic syndrome was shown to be an important contributor to worsening of memory among elderly women [36].

In conclusion, an increasing body of evidence suggests that disorders of glucose metabolism including diabetes, impaired fasting glucose and impaired glucose tolerance, as well as the cluster of risk factors known as metabolic syndrome are important predictors of cerebrovascular diseases, ischemic stroke, and accelerated cognitive decline and dementia. These findings carry important implications for preventive strategies for cerebrovascular disease and vascular cognitive impairment that are currently under investigation.

References

1   Warlow CP: Epidemiology of stroke. Lancet 1998;352(suppl 3):SIII1–SIII4.
2   Rothwell PM, Coull AJ, Silver LE, Fairhead JF, Giles MF, Lovelock CE, Redgrave JN, Bull LM, Welch SJ, Cuthbertson FC, Binney LE, Gutnikov SA, Anslow P, Banning AP, Mant D, Mehta Z: Population-based study of event-rate, incidence, case fatality, and mortality for all acute vascular events in all arterial territories (Oxford Vascular Study). Lancet 2005;366:1773–1783.
3   Tuomilehto J, Rastenyte D, Jousilahti P, Sarti C, Vartiainen E: Diabetes mellitus as a risk factor for death from stroke: prospective study of the middle-aged Finnish population. Stroke 1996;27: 210–215.
4   Folsom AR, Rasmussen ML, Chambless LE, Howard G, Cooper LS, Schmidt MI, Heiss G: Prospective associations of fasting insulin, body fat distribution, and diabetes with risk of ischemic stroke. The Atherosclerosis Risk In Communities (ARIC) study investigators. Diabetes Care 1999;22:1077–1083.
5   Stegmayr B, Asplund K: Diabetes as a risk factor for stroke: a population perspective. Diabetologia 1995;38:1061–1068.
6   Kuusisto J, Mykkanen L, Pyorala K, Laakso M: Non-insulin-dependent diabetes and its metabolic control are important predictors of stroke in elderly subjects. Stroke 1994;25:1157–1164.
7   Tuomilehto J, Rastenyte D: Diabetes and glucose intolerance as risk factors for stroke. J Cardiovasc Risk 1999;6:241–249.
8   Wannamethee SG, Perry IJ, Shaper AG: Nonfasting serum glucose and insulin concentrations and the risk of stroke. Stroke 1999;30:1780–1786.
9   Tanne D, Yaari S, Goldbourt U: Risk profile and prediction of long-term ischemic stroke mortality: a 21-year follow-up in the Israeli Ischemic Heart Disease (IIHD) Project. Circulation 1998;98:1365–1371.
10   Haffner SM, Lehto S, Ronnemaa T, Pyorala K, Laakso M: Mortality from coronary heart disease in subjects with type 2 diabetes and in nondiabetic subjects with and without prior myocardial infarction. N Engl J Med 1998;339:229–234.

11 Jorgensen H, Nakayama H, Raaschou HO, Olsen TS: Stroke in patients with diabetes. The Copenhagen Stroke Study. Stroke 1994;25:1977–1984.

12 You RX, McNeil JJ, O'Malley HM, Davis SM, Thrift AG, Donnan GA: Risk factors for stroke due to cerebral infarction in young adults. Stroke 1997;28:1913–1918.

13 Luchsinger JA, Tang MX, Stern Y, Shea S, Mayeux R: Diabetes mellitus and risk of Alzheimer's disease and dementia with stroke in a multiethnic cohort. Am J Epidemiol 2001;154:635–641.

14 Hankey GJ, Jamrozik K, Broadhurst RJ, Forbes S, Burvill PW, Anderson CS, Stewart-Wynne EG: Long-term risk of first recurrent stroke in the Perth Community Stroke Study. Stroke 1998;29: 2491–2500.

15 Tanne D, Koren-Morag N, Goldbourt U: Fasting plasma glucose and risk of incident ischemic stroke or transient ischemic attacks: a prospective cohort study. Stroke 2004;35:2351–2355.

16 Vermeer SE, Sandee W, Algra A, Koudstaal PJ, Kappelle LJ, Dippel DW: Impaired glucose tolerance increases stroke risk in nondiabetic patients with transient ischemic attack or minor ischemic stroke. Stroke 2006;37:1413–1417.

17 Kernan WN, Inzucchi SE, Viscoli CM, Brass LM, Bravata DM, Horwitz RI: Insulin resistance and risk for stroke. Neurology 2002;59:809–815.

18 Bravata DM, Wells CK, Kernan WN, Concato J, Brass LM, Gulanski BI: Association between impaired insulin sensitivity and stroke. Neuroepidemiology 2005;25:69–74.

19 Kernan WN, Viscoli CM, Inzucchi SE, Brass LM, Bravata DM, Shulman GI, McVeety JC: Prevalence of abnormal glucose tolerance following a transient ischemic attack or ischemic stroke. Arch Intern Med 2005;165:227–233.

20 Kernan WN, Inzucchi SE, Viscoli CM, Brass LM, Bravata DM, Shulman GI, McVeety JC, Horwitz RI: Pioglitazone improves insulin sensitivity among nondiabetic patients with a recent transient ischemic attack or ischemic stroke. Stroke 2003;34:1431–1436.

21 Koren-Morag N, Goldbourt U, Tanne D: Relation between the metabolic syndrome and ischemic stroke or transient ischemic attack: a prospective cohort study in patients with atherosclerotic cardiovascular disease. Stroke 2005;36:1366–1371.

22 Kurl S, Laukkanen JA, Niskanen L, Laaksonen D, Sivenius J, Nyyssonen K, Salonen JT: Metabolic syndrome and the risk of stroke in middle-aged men. Stroke 2006;37:806–811.

23 Chen HJ, Bai CH, Yeh WT, Chiu HC, Pan WH: Influence of metabolic syndrome and general obesity on the risk of ischemic stroke. Stroke 2006;37:1060–1064.

24 Schillaci G, Pirro M, Vaudo G, Gemelli F, Marchesi S, Porcellati C, Mannarino E: Prognostic value of the metabolic syndrome in essential hypertension. J Am Coll Cardiol 2004;43:1817–1822.

25 Iso H, Sato S, Kitamura A, Imano H, Kiyama M, Yamagishi K, Cui R, Tanigawa T, Shimamoto T: Metabolic syndrome and the risk of ischemic heart disease and stroke among Japanese men and women. Stroke 2007;38:1744–1751.

26 Tanne D, Koren-Morag N, Graff E, Goldbourt U: Blood lipids and first-ever ischemic stroke/transient ischemic attack in the Bezafibrate Infarction Prevention (BIP) Registry: high triglycerides constitute an independent risk factor. Circulation 2001;104:2892–2897.

27 Tanne D, Haim M, Boyko V, Goldbourt U, Reshef T, Matetzky S, Adler Y, Mekori YA, Behar S: Soluble intercellular adhesion molecule-1 and risk of future ischemic stroke: a nested case-control study from the Bezafibrate Infarction Prevention (BIP) Study cohort. Stroke 2002;33:2182–2186.

28 Tanne D, Benderly M, Goldbourt U, Haim M, Tenenbaum A, Fisman EZ, Matas Z, Adler Y, Zimmlichman R, Behar S: C-reactive protein as a predictor of incident ischemic stroke among patients with preexisting cardiovascular disease. Stroke 2006;37:1720–1724.

29 Tanne D, Yaari S, Goldbourt U: High-density lipoprotein cholesterol and risk of ischemic stroke mortality: a 21-year follow-up of 8586 men from the Israeli Ischemic Heart Disease Study. Stroke 1997;28:83–87.

30 Tanne D, Medalie JH, Goldbourt U: Body fat distribution and long-term risk of stroke mortality. Stroke 2005;36:1021–1025.

31 Najarian RM, Sullivan LM, Kannel WB, Wilson PW, D'Agostino RB, Wolf PA: Metabolic syndrome compared with type 2 diabetes mellitus as a risk factor for stroke: The Framingham Offspring Study. Arch Intern Med 2006;166:106–111.

32 Biessels GJ, Staekenborg S, Brunner E, Brayne C, Scheltens P: Risk of dementia in diabetes mellitus: a systematic review. Lancet Neurol 2006;5:64–74.

33 Schnaider Beeri M, Goldbourt U, Silverman JM, Noy S, Schmeidler J, Ravona-Springer R, Sverdlick A, Davidson M: Diabetes mellitus in midlife and the risk of dementia three decades later. Neurology 2004;63:1902–1907.

34 Abbatecola AM, Paolisso G, Lamponi M, Bandinelli S, Lauretani F, Launer L, Ferrucci L: Insulin resistance and executive dysfunction in older persons. J Am Geriatr Soc 2004;52:1713–1718.

35 Qiu WQ, Price LL, Hibberd P, Buell J, Collins L, Leins D, Mwamburi DM, Rosenberg I, Smaldone L, Scott TM, Siegel RD, Summergrad P, Sun X, Wagner C, Wang L, Yee J, Tucker KL, Folstein M: Executive dysfunction in homebound older people with diabetes mellitus. J Am Geriatr Soc 2006;54:496–501.

36 Komulainen P, Lakka TA, Kivipelto M, Hassinen M, Helkala EL, Haapala I, Nissinen A, Rauramaa R: Metabolic syndrome and cognitive function: a population-based follow-up study in elderly women. Dement Geriatr Cogn Disord 2007;23:29–34.

Prof. David Tanne, MD
Stroke Center, Department of Neurology Sheba Medical Center
Tel-Hashomer, and Division of Epidemiology and Preventive Medicine
Sackler Faculty of Medicine, Tel-Aviv University
Tel-Hashomer 52621 (Israel)
Tel. +972 3 520 2069, Fax +972 3 530 5791, E-Mail tanne@post.tau.ac.il

Fisman EZ, Tenenbaum A (eds): Cardiovascular Diabetology: Clinical, Metabolic and Inflammatory
Facets. Adv Cardiol. Basel, Karger, 2008, vol 45, pp 114–126

Impact of Metabolic Syndrome in Patients with Acute Coronary Syndrome

Micha S. Feinberg[a]   *Roseline Schwartz*[b]   *Solomon Behar*[b]

[a]Heart Institute and [b]Neufeld Cardiac Research Institute, Sheba Medical Center,
Tel-Hashomer, Sackler Faculty of Medicine, Tel-Aviv University, Tel-Aviv, Israel

Abstract

The reported incidence of metabolic syndrome among patients with an acute coronary syndrome varies between 29 and 46%. The standard fasting cut-off levels for glucose and blood pressure cannot be applied on admission in patients with acute coronary syndrome and therefore modified criteria were used to define the metabolic syndrome. Patients with metabolic syndrome and acute coronary syndrome had increased incidence of heart failure, and worse long-term mortality compared to those without metabolic syndrome. However, they had less heart failure than those with known diabetes mellitus. Hyperglycemia as a risk factor for poor outcome is particularly significant in patients with metabolic syndrome. De novo identification of the metabolic syndrome on admission has the potential to improve risk stratification and management of patients with an acute coronary syndrome.

Patients with metabolic syndrome have an increase risk of developing type 2 diabetes mellitus, cardiovascular disease, and long-term cardiovascular and overall mortality [1, 2]. The aim of this review is to summarize current published evidence of the impact of metabolic syndrome on the outcome of acute coronary syndrome as described recently in a few retrospective studies including the ACSIS 2004 (Acute Coronary Syndrome Israeli Survey) [3–7]. ACSIS is a national survey held once every 2 years and includes all patients admitted with an acute coronary syndrome to all coronary care units operating in Israel during a 2-month period.

The reported incidence of metabolic syndrome among patients with an acute coronary syndrome varies between 29 and 46% [3–7]. In studies where

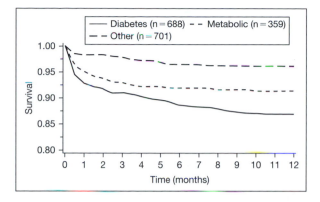

Fig. 1. Kaplan-Meier survival curve: patients with diabetes, metabolic syndrome and others (ACSIS 2004). p (log-rank) = 0.001.

patients with known diabetes mellitus were excluded from the analysis, the range was between 29 and 34% [3, 6] while it was between 38 and 46% [4, 5, 7] in those studies where diabetic patients were not excluded. In addition, significant differences exist regarding the definition of metabolic syndrome criteria, time intervals between the acute coronary syndrome and inclusion point, as well as duration of follow-up. Despite these diversities, patients with metabolic syndrome were consistently shown to have an increased rate of in-hospital complications [4, 6, 8] and worse long-term mortality [3–7].

Diabetes Mellitus vs. Metabolic Syndrome

Patients with diabetes mellitus have increased incidence of coronary artery disease and myocardial infarction with higher rates of mortality and morbidity [9–11]. In addition, patients with diabetes mellitus had worse outcome when compared with patients with metabolic syndrome (without known diabetes mellitus) and recent myocardial infarction [3], or acute coronary syndrome (fig. 1). It appears that the in-hospital course in patients with diabetes mellitus admitted with acute coronary syndrome as well as their demographic and history of coronary artery disease characteristics varies significantly from those with metabolic syndrome who resemble patients without diabetes mellitus excluding the determinants used to define metabolic syndrome (table 1). Therefore, in order to show the clear impact of metabolic syndrome on the outcome of patients with acute coronary syndrome those with diabetes mellitus should better be excluded [3, 6] (table 2).

Table 1. Patients' characteristics and outcome (ACSIS 2004)

Variable	DM (n = 688)	MS (n = 359)	Others (n = 701)	P1	P2
Age, years	66 ± 12	63 ± 13	62 ± 13	0.12	<0.001
Women	242 (35%)	98 (27%)	130 (19%)	0.001	0.01
Body mass index	28.2 ± 4.7	29.4 ± 4.2	25.3 ± 3.3	<0.001	<0.001
Hypertension	472 (69%)	275 (77%)	216 (31%)	<0.001	<0.001
Hyperlipidemia	412 (60%)	197 (55%)	279 (40%)	<0.001	0.007
Smoker (current)	151 (22%)	145 (40%)	313 (45%)	0.19	0.12
Past MI	257 (37%)	71 (20%)	147 (21%)	0.65	<0.001
Past angina pectoris	245 (36%)	106 (30%)	182 (26%)	0.22	<0.001
Past CABG	109 (16%)	33 (9%)	50 (7%)	0.24	<0.05
Past PCI	190 (28%)	63 (18%)	122 (17%)	0.95	0.003
Past heart failure	91 (13%)	13 (4%)	24 (3%)	0.87	<0.001
Chronic renal failure	105 (15%)	24 (7%)	33 (5%)	0.18	<0.001
Past stroke	76 (11%)	30 (8%)	36 (5%)	0.04	<0.001
Past PVD	80 (12%)	19 (5%)	28 (4%)	0.33	0.17
Malignancy	28 (4%)	13 (4%)	28 (4%)	0.77	0.72
Killip 2	134 (19%)	43 (21%)	70 (10%)		
Killip 3	78 (11%)	22 (6%)	23 (3%)		
Killip 4	8 (1%)	2 (1%)	5 (1%)		
Killip on admission ≥2	220 (31%)	67 (19%)	98 (14%)	0.03	0.001
Admission systolic blood pressure, mm Hg	147 ± 31	146 ± 31	138 ± 29	<0.001	0.64
Admission diastolic blood pressure, mm Hg	81 ± 17	84 ± 17	81 ± 17	0.003	0.026
Glucose on admission, mg/dl	243 ± 106	156 ± 62	121 ± 35	<0.001	<0.001
Triglycerides, mg/dl	200 ± 311	202 ± 113	127 ± 92	<0.001	0.94
HDL, mg/dl	41 ± 18	36 ± 9	46 ± 13	<0.001	<0.001
LVEF, %[1]	43 ± 12	47 ± 12	47 ± 11	0.56	<0.001

ACS					
Q wave MI	243 (35%)	168 (47%)	338 (48%)		
Non-Q-wave MI	245 (35%)	114 (32%)	199 (28%)		
Unstable angina	205 (30%)	77 (21%)	164 (23%)	0.49	0.001
MI location					
Anterior	194 (28%)	123 (34%)	245 (35%)	0.82	0.04
Inferior	188 (27%)	114 (32%)	205 (30%)	0.52	0.13

Others = Patients without metabolic syndrome (MS) or clinically diagnosed diabetes mellitus (DM); available in 72% of patients. MI = Myocardial infarction; CABG = coronary artery bypass grafting; PCI = percutaneous coronary intervention; PVD = peripheral vascular disease; HDL = high-density lipoproteins cholesterol; LVEF = left ventricular ejection fraction; ACS = acute coronary syndrome. P1 = MS vs. others, P2 = DM vs. MS.

[1]Available for 70% of patients.

Table 2. Hospital complications and outcome (ACSIS 2004)

Variable	DM (n = 688)	MS (n = 359)	Others (n = 701)	P1	P2
CHF (all)	134 (19.5%)	50 (13.9%)	66 (9.4%)	0.03	0.03
Stroke	6 (0.9%)	5 (1.4%)	1 (0.1%)	0.01	0.53
Renal failure	67 (9.7%)	19 (5.3%)	23 (3.3%)	0.11	0.13
Renal MI	8 (1.2%)	4 (1.1%)	6 (0.9%)	0.68	0.94
7 days' mortality	23 (3.3%)	8 (2.2%)	7 (1.0%)	0.11	0.32
30 days' mortality	49 (7.1%)	18 (5.0%)	12 (1.7%)	0.002	0.19
6 months' mortality	79 (11.5%)	29 (8.1%)	25 (3.6%)	0.002	0.09
1-year mortality	102 (14.8%)	32 (8.9%)	32 (4.6%)	0.001	0.07

Others = Patients without metabolic syndrome (MS) or clinically diagnosed diabetes mellitus (DM).
Abbreviations as in table 1.
P1 = MS vs. others, P2 = DM vs. MS.

Definition of Metabolic Syndrome in Acute Coronary Syndrome (table 3)

Early determination whether a patient has metabolic syndrome is desirable as it effects early outcome [6, 8]. The standard NCEP ATP III definition of metabolic syndrome is based on detection of 3 of 5 components in a stable fasting condition; impaired glucose metabolism, hypertension, decreased HDL cholesterol, increased triglycerides and obesity [12]. The standard fasting cut-off levels for glucose and blood pressure cannot be applied at admission in patients with acute coronary syndrome and therefore current publications have defined metabolic syndrome in the context of acute coronary syndrome in different ways. Zeller et al. [4] and Nakatani et al. [7] used pre-discharge assessment for this purpose and Schwartz et al. [5] used history of diabetes and hypertension instead of assessment of blood pressure and fasting glucose levels.

It should be noted that in the absence of diabetes, nonfasting blood glucose level generally is not >140 mg/dl [13]. We therefore used blood glucose level >140 mg/dl (increased occasional glucose) as a criterion for impaired glucose metabolism on admission of patients with acute coronary syndrome [6] (ACSIS 2004).

Hypotension is a marker of high-risk patients admitted with acute coronary syndrome, reflecting pump failure. Higher blood pressure levels were identified as protective in such a population [14]. Mild elevations of blood pressure

Table 3. Definition of metabolic syndrome in the studies reporting outcome OF acute coronary syndrome

NCEP ATP III[1]	Zeller et al. [4]	Schwartz et al. [5]	Feinberg et al. [6]	Nakatani et al. [7]
Elevated fasting glucose: ≥100 mg/dl	Pre-discharge fasting glucose ≥100 mg/dl	History of diabetes mellitus	Glucose on admission >140 mg/dl	Pre-discharge fasting blood glucose >110 mg/dl or antidiabetic therapy
Elevated blood pressure: ≥130/85 mm Hg	Pre-discharge blood pressure ≥130/85 mm Hg (cardiogenic shock excluded)	History of hypertension or blood pressure ≥130/85 mm Hg	History of hypertension	Pre-discharge blood pressure ≥130 mm Hg, ≥85 mm Hg, or use of antihypertensive therapy
Reduced HDL men <40 mg/dl women <50 mg/dl	Reduced HDL men <40 mg/dl women <50 mg/dl	Reduced HDL men <40 mg/dl women <50 mg/dl	Reduced HDL men <40 mg/dl women <50 mg/dl	Pre-discharge reduced HDL men <40 mg/dl women <50 mg/dl
Elevated triglycerides ≥150 mg/dl	Elevated triglycerides ≥150 mg/dl	Elevated triglycerides ≥150 mg/dl	Elevated triglycerides ≥150 mg/dl	Pre-discharge elevated triglycerides ≥150 mg/dl
Elevated waist circumference men ≥102 cm women ≥88 cm	Waist circumference men ≥102 cm women ≥88 cm	BMI >30	BMI >28	Pre-discharge BMI >25

[1]The Third Report of The National Cholesterol Education Program (NCEP) Expert Panel on Detection, JAMA 2001;285:2486–2497.

probably reflect a normal physiologic response in the context of acute coronary syndrome. To avoid this pitfall, we used a preexisting diagnosis of hypertension as the criterion for metabolic syndrome [6]. Serum lipids (HDL cholesterol and triglycerides) are expected to change less early at admission [15], and those criteria were not modified. Increased BMI is used as a criterion for obesity when waist circumference is not available [16]; however, different cut-off levels were proposed for this purpose. Nakatani et al. [7] used 25 for a Japanese population, Schwartz et al. [5] used 30, and 28 was used in the ACSIS 2004.

In-Hospital Complications in Patients with Metabolic Syndrome

Patients with metabolic syndrome and acute coronary syndrome had increased incidence of heart failure on admission and during hospitalization, requiring more frequent mechanical ventilation, compared to those without metabolic syndrome [6]. However, they had less heart failure than those with known diabetes mellitus (tables 1, 2). Clavijo et al. [8] also found an increased incidence of heart failure among patients with acute coronary syndrome and metabolic syndrome undergoing coronary angiography without excluding those with diabetes mellitus.

The incidence of stroke was significantly higher among patients with metabolic syndrome in ACSIS 2004 [6]; however, the number of patients with this complication was small (table 2). Zeller et al. [4] did not report a higher rate of stroke among patients with metabolic syndrome. Clavijo et al. [8] reported a high incidence of renal failure among patients with metabolic syndrome that had a coronary angiography. The rate of recurrent myocardial infarction was similar among those with metabolic syndrome compared to others and patients with diabetes mellitus [4, 6] (table 2).

Hyperglycemia with Metabolic Syndrome

An independent graded association between increasing levels of admission glucose and adverse clinical outcomes was reported in patients with an acute myocardial infarction [17]. Hyperglycemia in patients with an acute coronary syndrome is consistently associated with increased mortality and heart failure [17–19]. The incidence of hyperglycemia is higher among patients with metabolic syndrome, and the early outcome of patients with hyperglycemia and metabolic syndrome is worse than in those without hyperglycemia [6]. In the ACSIS 2004, most patients who died at 30 days (74%) had glucose levels >140 mg/dl and most (85%) had metabolic syndrome [6]. The impact of metabolic syndrome on 30 days' mortality in patients with and without hyperglycemia on admission is shown in figure 2. Patients with metabolic syndrome and hyperglycemia on admission had more than a 3-fold increase of 30 days' mortality rate compared with patients with hyperglycemia but without metabolic syndrome (8.3 vs. 2.5%, $p < 0.05$) (fig. 2).

The exact means by which hyperglycemia confers an increase in cardiovascular risk in the setting of acute coronary syndrome is not completely understood. Several potential mechanisms have been proposed to explain the association between stress hyperglycemia on admission for acute coronary syndrome and increased early and late mortality [20–25]. Insulin deficiency is associated with increased lipolysis and excess fatty acids are toxic to the ischemic myocardium [20, 21]. Hyperglycemia may cause osmotic diuresis, volume depletion and reduced stroke volume, and may adversely effect coagulation [23], platelets [24], and endothelial function [25].

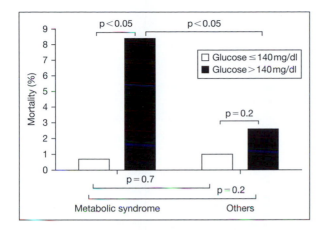

Fig. 2. Thirty days' mortality rate among non-clinically diagnosed diabetes mellitus patients with hyperglycemia (glucose >140 mg/dl) with and without metabolic syndrome.

Undiagnosed diabetes is common in patients hospitalized because of acute coronary syndrome [26]. Although the stressful situation of acute coronary syndrome leads to a nonspecific increase in plasma glucose, the real prevalence of undiagnosed diabetes and impaired glucose tolerance is reported to be high in patients with an acute coronary syndrome [27]. Furthermore, it has been shown that newly detected abnormal glucose tolerance in patients with an acute coronary syndrome is a strong predictor of future cardiovascular events [28].

These findings seem to indicate that the significance of hyperglycemia as a risk factor for poor outcome is particularly significant in patients with metabolic syndrome.

Outcome of Patients with Metabolic Syndrome with Acute Coronary Syndrome (table 4)

Levantesi et al. [3] described the impact of metabolic syndrome in a large multi-center study of patients with a recent myocardial infarction (<3 months, median; 16 days). This study showed that patients with metabolic syndrome without a history of diabetes mellitus had an increased 3.5-year mortality rate compared to patients with neither. Zeller et al. [4] found a significant association between metabolic syndrome and mortality in patients with acute myocardial

Table 4. Impact of metabolic syndrome on outcome of patients with acute or recent coronary syndromes

	Study population	n	MS (%)	Follow-up	End point	HR (95% CI)
Levantesi et al. [3]	post recent MI (up to 3 months, median 16 days)	10,384	29	1,260 days	all cause mortality 14.5 (diabetics) vs. 8.5 (MS) vs. 7.4% (others)	1.29 (1.10–1.51)
Zeller et al. [4]	post acute MI	633	46	hospitalization	all cause mortality 10.7 vs. 3.8%	nonsignificant after adjustment
Schwartz et al. [5]	ACS	3,038	38*	16 weeks	death, nonfatal MI, cardiac arrest or UA 19 vs. 14%	1.49 (1.24–1.79)
Feinberg et al. [6]	ACS non-diabetics	1,060	34	1 year	all cause mortality 8.9 vs. 4.6%	1.96 (1.18–3.24) adjusted
Nakatani et al. [7]	post acute MI	3,858	43	725 days (median)	cardiac death or nonfatal MI 7.2 vs. 5.4%	1.48 (1.13–1.94) adjusted

MS = Metabolic syndrome; HR = hazard ratio; CI = confidence interval; ACS = acute coronary syndrome; UN = unstable angina.
*MS is defined as 3 of the following: history of diabetes, history of hypertension or blood pressure ≥130/≥85 mm Hg, BMI >30, HDL >40 mg% (men) or >50 mg% (women), triglycerides >150 mg%.

infarction without excluding diabetics. In the Myocardial Ischemia Reduction with Aggressive Cholesterol Lowering (MIRACLE) trial, patients with acute coronary syndrome and metabolic syndrome (including patients with diabetes) had increased all-cause mortality and an increased primary end point (death, nonfatal myocardial infarction, cardiac arrest, or recurrent unstable myocardial ischemia) during a 16-week follow-up [5]. In the ACSIS 2004, metabolic syndrome was a significant independent risk factor for 1-year all-cause mortality after adjustment for age, gender, Killip on admission and other risks associated with mortality that were present on admission in patients with acute coronary syndrome without clinically diagnosed diabetes mellitus [6]. Nakatani et al. [7] reported an increased rate of cardiac death or nonfatal myocardial infarction among patients with metabolic syndrome (without excluding diabetics) during a 2-year follow-up period (median).

Criteria for the presence of metabolic syndrome were prospectively collected in the Acute Coronary Syndrome Israeli Survey (ACSIS 2006) for 1,153 non-clinically diagnosed diabetes mellitus patients. Fasting glucose levels were determined the day following admission using standard NCEP ATP III cut-off levels and waist circumference was measured on admission. The 30 days' mortality rate among patients with metabolic syndrome was significantly higher than in patients without clinically diagnosed diabetes mellitus or metabolic syndrome (3.8 vs. 1.6%, p = 0.02) [unpubl. data]. Metabolic syndrome remained a significant risk factor for 30 days' mortality with an odds ratio (95% CI) of 2.49 (1.06–6.57) after adjustment for age, gender and Killip >1 on admission.

Potential Mechanisms Involved with Acute Coronary Syndrome in Patients with Metabolic Syndrome

In addition to the traditional cardiovascular risk factors (dyslipidemia, obesity, hypertension and hyperglycemia), there are a number of nontraditional risk factors in people with metabolic syndrome. These include first of all insulin resistance and hyperinsulinemia [12], which may confer some additional independent risk. Insulin resistance is associated with increased lipolysis and excess fatty acids toxic to the ischemic myocardium [20, 21]. Additional nontraditional risk factors include increases in oxidative stress, angiotensin II effects, and markers of inflammation (increase of interleukin-6, tumor necrosis factor-α, C-reactive protein, plasminogen activator inhibitor-1 and leptin, and reduced adiponectin levels) [29]. All these combine to increase atherogenesis, endothelial dysfunction and inflammation in people with metabolic syndrome before and after an acute coronary event.

Clinical Implications

Patients with metabolic syndrome have an increased incidence of congestive heart failure during hospitalization and an augmented mortality rate that persists for over 1 year. Early de novo identification of metabolic syndrome on admission using modified NCEP ATP III criteria is feasible even in the nonfasting and stressful situation generally associated with an acute coronary syndrome. Hyperglycemia is a common marker of increased risk in patients with metabolic syndrome. Patients with metabolic syndrome have less established coronary artery disease, diastolic dysfunction and heart failure than diabetics and they might benefit from early aggressive risk reduction. Based on these findings, we believe that de novo identification metabolic syndrome on admission has the potential to improve risk stratification and management of patients with an acute coronary syndrome. However, caution should be used in interpreting these finding since they were identified retrospectively.

References

1   Lakka HM, Laaksonen DE, Lakka TA, Niskanen LK, Kumpusalo E, Tuomilehto JT, Salonen JT: The metabolic syndrome an total and cardiovascular disease mortality in middle aged men. JAMA 2002;288:2709–2016.
2   Grundy SM, Cleeman JI, Daniels SR, Donato KA, Eckel RH, Franklin BA, Gordon DJ, Krauss RM, Savage PJ, Smith SC Jr, Spertus JA, Costa F: Diagnosis and management of the metabolic syndrome: an American Heart Association/National Heart, Lung, and Blood Institute Scientific Statement. Circulation 2005;112:2735–2752.
3   Levantesi, Macchia A, Marfisi R, Franzosi MG, Maggioni AP, Nicolosi GL, Schweiger C, Tavazzi L, Tognoni G, Valagussa F, Marchioli R, on behalf of the GISSI-Prevenzione Investigators: Metabolic syndrome and risk of cardiovascular events after myocardial infarction. J Am Coll Cardiol 2005;46:277–283.
4   Zeller M, Steg PG, Ravisy J, Laurent Y, Janin-Manificat L, L'Huillier I, Beer JC, Oudot A, Rioufol G, Makki H, Farnier M, Rochette L, Vergès B, Cottin Y, for the Observatoire des Infarctus de Côte-d'Or Survey Working Group: Prevalence and impact of metabolic syndrome on hospital outcomes in acute myocardial infarction. Arch Intern Med 2005;165:1192–1198.
5   Schwartz GG, Szarek M, Olsson AG, Sasiela WJ: Relation of characteristics of metabolic syndrome to short term prognosis and effects of statin therapy after acute coronary syndrome. Diabetes Care 2005;28:2508–2013.
6   Feinberg MS, Schwartz R, Tanne D, Fisman EZ, Hod H, Zahger D, Schwammethal E, Eldar M, Behar S, Tenenbaum A: Impact of the metabolic syndrome on the clinical outcomes of non-clinically diagnosed diabetic patients with acute coronary syndrome. Am J Cardiol 2007;99: 667–672.
7   Nakatani D, Sakata Y, Hiroshi Sato H, Mizuno H, Masahiko Shimizu M, Suna S, Ito H, Koretsune Y, Hirayama A, Hori M, on behalf of the Osaka Acute Coronary Insufficiency Study (OACIS) Group: Clinical impact of metabolic syndrome and its additive effect with smoking on subsequent cardiac events after acute myocardial infarction. Am J Cardiol 2007;99:885–889.
8   Clavijo LC, Pinto TL, Kuchulakanti PK, Torguson R, Chu WW, Satler LF, Kent KM, Suddath WO, Pichard AD, Waksman R: Metabolic syndrome in patients with acute myocardial infarction is associated with increased infarct size and in-hospital complications. Cardiovasc Revascular Med 2006;7:7–11.

9 Stone PH, Muller JE, Hartwell T, York BJ, Rutherford JD, Parker CB, Turi ZG, Strauss HW, Willerson JT, Robertson T, et al: The effect of diabetes mellitus on prognosis and serial left ventricular function after acute myocardial infarction: contribution of both coronary disease and diastolic left ventricular dysfunction to the adverse prognosis. The MILIS Study Group. J Am Coll Cardiol 1989;14:49–57.

10 Herlitz J, Malmberg K, Karlson BW, Rydén L, Hjalmarson A: Mortality and morbidity during a five-year follow-up of diabetics with myocardial infarction. Acta Med Scand 1988;224:31–38.

11 Woods KL, Samanta A, Burden AC: Diabetes mellitus as a risk factor for acute myocardial infarction in Asians and Europeans. Br Heart J 1989;62:118–122.

12 Grundy SM, Brewer HB Jr, Cleeman JI, Smith SC Jr, Lenfant C, American Heart Association, National Heart, Lung, and Blood Institute: Definition of MS: report of the National Heart, Lung, and Blood Institute/American Heart Association conference on scientific issues related to definition. Circulation 2004;109:433–438.

13 American Diabetes Association Consensus Statement: Postprandial blood glucose. Diabetes Care 2001;24;775–778.

14 Jonas M, Grossman E, Boyko V, Behar S, Hod H, Reicher-Reiss H: Relation of early and one-year outcome after acute myocardial infarction to systemic arterial blood pressure on admission. Am J Cardiol 1999;84:162–165.

15 Henkin Y, Crystal E, Goldberg Y, Friger M, Lorber J, Zuili I, Shany S: Usefulness of lipoprotein changes during acute coronary syndromes for predicting post-discharge lipoprotein levels. Am J Cardiol 2002;89:7–11.

16 Tenenbaum A, Motro M, Fisman EZ, Tanne D, Boyko V, Behar S: Bezafibrate for the secondary prevention of myocardial infarction in patients with MS. Arch Intern Med 2005;165:1154–1160.

17 Svensson AM, McGuire DK, Abrahamsson P, Dellborg M: Association between hyper- and hypoglycaemia and 2 year all-cause mortality risk in diabetic patients with acute coronary events. Eur Heart J 2005;26:1255–1261.

18 Stranders I, Diamant M, van Gelder RE, Spruijt HJ, Twisk JWR, Heine RJ, Visser FC: Admission blood glucose level as risk indicator of death after myocardial infarction in patients with and without diabetes mellitus. Arch Intern Med 2004;164:982–988.

19 Grundy SM: Metabolic syndrome: connecting and reconciling cardiovascular and diabetes worlds. J Am Coll Cardiol 2006;47:1093–1100.

20 Tansey MJ, Opie LH: Relation between plasma free fatty acids and arrhythmias within the first twelve hours of acute myocardial infarction. Lancet 1983;ii:419–422.

21 Oliver MF, Opie LH: Effects of glucose and fatty acids on myocardial ischaemia and arrhythmias. Lancet 1994;343:155–158.

22 Tansey MJ, Opie LH: Plasma glucose on admission to hospital as a metabolic index of the severity of acute myocardial infarction. Can J Cardiol 1986;2:326–331.

23 Davi G, Catalano I, Averna M, Notarbartolo A, Strano A, Ciabattoni G, Patrono C: Thromboxane biosynthesis and platelet function in type II diabetes mellitus. N Engl J Med 1990;322:1769–1774.

24 Jain SK, Nagi DK, Slavin BM, Lumb PJ, Yudkin JS: Insulin therapy in type 2 diabetic subjects suppresses plasminogen activator inhibitor (PAI-1) activity and proinsulin-like molecules independently of glycaemic control. Diabet Med 1993;10:27–32.

25 Williams SB, Goldfine AB, Timimi FK, Ting HH, Roddy MA, Simonson DC, Creager MA: Acute hyperglycemia attenuates endothelium-dependent vasodilation in humans in vivo. Circulation 1998;97:1695–1701.

26 Norhammar A, Tenerz A, Nilsson G, Hamsten A, Efendic S, Rydén L, Malmberg K: Glucose metabolism in patients with acute myocardial infarction and no previous diagnosis of diabetes mellitus: a prospective study. Lancet 2002;359:2140–2144.

27 Bartnik M, Rydén L, Ferrari R, Malmberg K, Pyörälä K, Simoons M, Standl E, Soler-Soler J, Ohrvik J, Euro Heart Survey Investigators: The prevalence of abnormal glucose regulation in patients with coronary artery disease across Europe: The Euro Heart Survey on Diabetes and the Heart. Eur Heart J 2004;25:1880–1890.

28 Bartnik M, Malmberg K, Norhammar A, Tenerz A, Ohrvik J, Rydén L: Newly detected abnormal glucose tolerance: an important predictor of long-term outcome after myocardial infarction. Eur Heart J 2004;25:1990–1997.

29 Salmenniemi U, Ruotsalainen E, Pihlajamaki J, Vauhkonen I, Kainulainen S, Punnonen K, Vanninen E, Laakso M: Multiple abnormalities in glucose and energy metabolism and coordinated changes in levels of adiponectin, cytokines, and adhesion molecules in subjects with metabolic syndrome. Circulation 2004;110:3842–3848.

Prof. Micha S. Feinberg, MD
Heart Institute, Sheba Medical Center
Tel-Hashomer 52621 (Israel)
Tel. +972 3 530 2433, Fax +972 3 530 2407, E-Mail micha.feinberg@sheba.health.gov.il

Fisman EZ, Tenenbaum A (eds): Cardiovascular Diabetology: Clinical, Metabolic and Inflammatory Facets. Adv Cardiol. Basel, Karger, 2008, vol 45, pp 127–153

. . . .

Optimal Management of Combined Dyslipidemia: What Have We Behind Statins Monotherapy?

Alexander Tenenbaum[a,b]   *Enrique Z. Fisman*[b]   *Michael Motro*[a]   *Yehuda Adler*[a]

[a]Cardiac Rehabilitation Institute, Chaim Sheba Medical Center, Tel-Hashomer, affiliated with the Sackler Faculty of Medicine, Tel-Aviv University, Tel-Aviv, [b]Cardiovascular Diabetology Research Foundation, Holon, Israel

Abstract

Evidence of the effectiveness of 3-hydroxy-3-methylglutaryl coenzyme A reductase inhibitors (statins) within continuum of atherothrombotic conditions and particularly in the treatment and prevention of coronary heart disease (CHD) is well established. Large-scale, randomized, prospective trials involving patients with CHD have shown that statins reduce the clinical consequences of atherosclerosis, including cardiovascular deaths, nonfatal myocardial infarction and stroke, hospitalization for acute coronary syndrome and heart failure, as well as the need for coronary revascularization. Direct testing of varying degrees of low-density lipoprotein (LDL)-cholesterol lowering has now been carried out in 4 large outcomes trials: PROVE IT–TIMI 22, A to Z, TNT and IDEAL. However, the question whether more aggressive LDL-cholesterol lowering by high-dose statins monotherapy is an appropriate strategy is still open: higher doses of statins are more effective mainly for the prevention of the nonfatal cardiovascular events but such doses are associated with an increase in hepatotoxicity, myopathy and concerns regarding noncardiovascular death. Moreover, despite the increasing use of statins, a significant number of coronary events still occur and many such events take place in patients presenting with type 2 diabetes and metabolic syndrome. More and more attention is now being paid to combined atherogenic dyslipidemia which typically presented in patients with type 2 diabetes and metabolic syndrome. This mixed dyslipidemia (or 'lipid quartet') – hypertriglyceridemia, low high-density lipoprotein (HDL)-cholesterol levels, a preponderance of small, dense LDL particles and an accumulation of cholesterol-rich remnant particles – emerged as the greatest 'competitor' of LDL-cholesterol among lipid risk factors for cardiovascular disease. Most recent extensions of the fibrates trials (BIP, HHS, VAHIT and FIELD) give further support to the hypothesis that patients with insulin-resistant syndromes such as diabetes and/or metabolic syndrome might be the ones to derive the most benefit from therapy with fibrates. However, different fibrates may have a somewhat different spectrum of effects. Other lipid-modifying strategies included using of niacin, ezetimibe, bile acid sequestrants, CETP inhibitors and omega–3 fatty acids. Particularly, ezetimibe/statins combinations provide superior lipid-modifying benefits compared with any statins monotherapy in patients with atherogenic dyslipidemia. Atherogenic dyslipidemia is associated with increased levels of chylomicrons and their remnants containing 3 main components: apolipoprotein B-48, triglycerides and cholesterol ester of intestinal origin. Reduction in accessibility for one of them (specifically cholesteryl ester lessening due to ezetimibe administration) could lead to a decrease of the entire production of chylomicrons and result in a decrease of the hepatic body triglycerides pool as confirmed in number of clinical studies. However, the ENHANCE study showed no difference in the progression of carotid atherosclerosis between ezetimibe/simvastatin vs. simvastatin alone over a 2-year period. Conclusions regarding ezetimibe/statins combinations should not be made until the three large clinical outcome trials will be completed within the next 2–3 years. In addition, bezafibrate as a pan-PPAR activator has clearly demonstrated beneficial pleiotropic effects related to glucose metabolism, insulin sensitivity and pancreatic beta cell protection. Because fibrates, niacin, ezetimibe, omega–3 fatty acids and statins each regulate serum lipids by different mechanisms, combination therapy – selected on the basis of their safety and effectiveness, could be more helpful in achieving a comprehensive lipid control as compared with statins monotherapy.

Introduction

The evidence of the effectiveness of 3-hydroxy-3-methylglutaryl coenzyme A reductase inhibitors (statins) within continuum of atherothrombotic conditions and particularly in the treatment and prevention of coronary heart disease (CHD) is well established. Large-scale, randomized, prospective trials involving patients with CHD have shown that statins reduce the clinical consequences of atherosclerosis, including cardiovascular deaths, nonfatal myocardial infarction and stroke, hospitalization for acute coronary syndrome and heart failure, as well as the need for coronary revascularization [1–8].

However, despite the increasing use of statins, a significant number of coronary events still occur and many such events take place in patients presenting with type 2 diabetes and metabolic syndrome. More and more attention is now being paid to combined atherogenic dyslipidemia which typically presented in patients with type 2 diabetes and metabolic syndrome [9]. This mixed dyslipidemia (or 'lipid quartet') – hypertriglyceridemia, low high-density lipoprotein-cholesterol (HDL-C) levels, a preponderance of small, dense low-density lipoprotein-cholesterol (LDL-C) particles and an accumulation of cholesterol-rich remnant particles (e.g. high levels of apolipoprotein B) – emerged as the greatest 'competitor' of LDL-C among lipid risk factors for cardiovascular disease.

Therapeutic approach involves intervention at a macro-level and control of multiple risk factors using therapeutic lifestyle approaches (diet control and increased physical activity, pharmacotherapy – anti-obesity agents) for control of obesity and visceral obesity, and a targeted approach for the control of individual risk factors. Anti-obesity drugs such as sibutramine, orlistat and rimonabant appear promising in this regard. The lifestyle changes recommended by NCEP ATP III for controlling dyslipidemia (i.e. elevated levels of triglycerides and decreased levels of HDL-C in patients with metabolic syndrome or type 2 DM include (1) reduced intake of saturated fats and dietary cholesterol, (2) intake of dietary options to enhance lowering of LDL-C, (3) weight control, and (4) increased physical activity. If lifestyle changes are not successful for individuals at high risk of developing CHD, or for those who currently have CHD, a CHD risk equivalent, or persistent atherogenic dyslipidemia, then pharmacotherapy may be necessary. Current therapeutic use of statins as monotherapy even in optimal doses and achieved target LDL-C reduction is still leaving many patients with mixed atherogenic dyslipidemia at high risk for coronary events. Moreover, the question whether more aggressive LDL-C lowering by high-dose statins monotherapy is an appropriate strategy is still open: higher doses of statins are more effective mainly for the prevention of the nonfatal cardiovascular events but such doses are associated with an increase in hepatotoxicity, myopathy and concerns regarding noncardiovascular death [8].

Targeting multiple lipid pathways can provide greater reductions in LDL-C as well as improvements in other lipid parameters. In the current chapter, we briefly examine recent data regarding different lipid-lowering approaches (statins as monotherapy, non-statins-based or combined strategies) in patients with mixed atherogenic dyslipidemia.

Intensive LDL-C-Lowering Strategy Using Statins as Monotherapy

Direct testing of varying degrees of LDL-C lowering has now been carried out in 4 large outcomes trials: PROVE IT–TIMI 22, A to Z, TNT and IDEAL. The fifth and largest of the trials comparing intensive vs. standard-dose statins therapy, the Study of the Effectiveness of Additional Reductions in Cholesterol and Homocysteine (SEARCH), is expected to report its findings in 2007, comparing simvastatin 80 mg daily vs. simvastatin 20 mg daily among 12,064 patients with a previous myocardial infarction (MI). The 'scores' of the already completed trials where 'positive' means 'in favor of intensive LDL-C-lowering strategy using statins as monotherapy' are as follows:

First, the Pravastatin or Atorvastatin Evaluation and Infection Treatment-Thrombolysis in Myocardial Infarction (PROVE IT–TIMI 22) trial. This trial compared a standard-dose pravastatin that achieved a median LDL-C level of 95 mg/dl, with a more intensive strategy using high-dose atorvastatin that achieved a median LDL-C level of 62 mg/dl. The trial results demonstrated a statistically significant benefit of the more intensive statins treatment, with a 16% reduction in the risk of death and major cardiovascular events, which emerged rapidly and was observed over the subsequent 2 years following an acute coronary syndrome [2].

Second, the A to Z trial compared early intensive (40 mg/day of simvastatin for 1 month followed by 80 mg/day thereafter, n = 2,265) versus a delayed conservative strategy (receiving placebo for 4 months followed by 20 mg/day of simvastatin, n = 2,232) in patients with acute coronary syndromes [3]. It was a negative study which did not achieve the prespecified end point. However, the early initiation of an aggressive simvastatin regimen resulted in a favorable trend toward reduction of major cardiovascular events, but outcomes were not statistically significant.

Third, the Treating to New Targets (TNT) trial had a highly significant reduction in cardiovascular events and expanded the benefit of more intensive statins therapy to patients with stable coronary artery disease. There were reductions in cardiovascular death, myocardial infarction (MI), need for revascularization, and stroke with use of high-dose vs. standard-dose atorvastatin [4]. Although the trial results were consistent with the concept that for cholesterol, 'the lower the better', concerns were raised regarding a nonsignificant difference in total and noncardiovascular death in favor of less intensive statins therapy.

Fourth, the Incremental Decrease in End Points Through Aggressive Lipid Lowering (IDEAL) trial was a prospective, randomized, open-label, blinded end-point evaluation trial with a median follow-up of 4.8 years, which enrolled 8,888 patients aged 80 years or younger with a history of acute MI. Patients were randomly assigned to receive a high dose of atorvastatin (80 mg/day; n = 4,439), or usual-dose simvastatin (20 mg/day; n = 4,449). Again, in this study of patients with previous MI, intensive lowering of LDL-C did not result in a significant reduction in the primary outcome of major coronary events. There were no differences in cardiovascular or all-cause mortality. Patients in the atorvastatin group had higher rates of drug discontinuation due to nonserious adverse events. However, when using the primary end point of the TNT and/or PROVE IT–TIMI 22 trials, which also included stroke and/or revascularization, there was a significant reduction of cardiovascular events rate: the primary differences were in the nonfatal end points [5]. Overall, the 4 trials of aggressive statins therapy to date have shown that the degree of LDL-C lowering was related to the degree of cardiovascular clinical benefit [7] but not to a total mortality reduction (in expense of nonsignificant trends in noncardiovascular causes of deaths). A new meta-analysis of these four trials showed a significant reduction in coronary death or any cardiovascular event with intensive treatment [10]. A significant 16% odds reduction in coronary death or myocardial infarction (p < 0.00001), as well as a significant 16% odds reduction of coronary death or any cardiovascular event (p < 0.00001) in those receiving high-dose statins therapy versus standard dose were found. No difference was observed in total or noncardiovascular mortality, but a trend toward decreased cardiovascular mortality (odds reduction 12%, p = 0.054) was observed. It should be noted that meta-analysis as a statistical technique enjoyed considerable success in influencing medical opinion and treatment practice in selected areas. However, the level of evidence required for consensus is not well understood and cannot be defined precisely. The retrospective nature of meta-analysis and the risks of biased data acquisition mandate a conservative approach to data analysis and interpretation [10]. Meta-analysis can be used productively in planning new clinical trials, but it can not be a substitute for prospective randomized trials. Again, a meta-analysis of the four trials of intensive statins therapy still failed to detect a statistical difference in total mortality [11]. Although the increase in deaths from noncardiovascular causes in part of the trials could be due to chance, it is still a matter of concern. Any reduction in nonfatal events may be outweighed by more numerous and more severe adverse effects [12]. Because many nonfatal events resolve with little residual damage or discomfort, meticulous recording of all possible adverse side effects is mandatory.

Cholesterol is vital for the development and function of the brain. It is therefore unsurprising that reduced concentrations may produce mental and neurological complaints such as severe irritability, aggressive behavior, suicidal impulses, cognitive impairment, memory loss, global amnesia, polyneuropathy, and erectile dysfunction [13–20]. In many cases the symptoms were reversible and recurred after rechallenge. Compared with the low-dose statins therapy, intensive statins therapy has been associated with increased incidence of discontinuation, hepatotoxicity (0.2–1.1 vs. 0.9–3.3%, respectively) and myalgia (1.1–4.7 vs. 1.8–4.8%, respectively). It must be kept in mind that the incidence of side effects with the high-dose statins might be higher in clinical practice than that reported in these clinical trials due to careful selection of patients in these trials [21].

In accordance with AHA/ACC guidelines for secondary prevention for patients with coronary and other atherosclerotic vascular disease, when the LDL-C <70 mg/dl target is chosen, it may be prudent to increase statins therapy in a graded fashion to determine a patient's response and tolerance. Furthermore, if it is not possible to attain LDL-C <70 mg/dl because of a high baseline LDL-C, it generally is possible to achieve LDL-C reductions of >50% with either statins or LDL-C-lowering drug combinations. Moreover, this guideline for patients with atherosclerotic disease does not modify the recommendations of the 2004 ATP III update for patients without atherosclerotic disease who have diabetes or multiple risk factors and a 10-year risk level for CHD >20%. In the latter 2 types of high-risk patients, the recommended LDL-C goal of <100 mg/dl has not changed. Finally, to avoid any misunderstanding about cholesterol management in general, it must be emphasized that a reasonable cholesterol level of <70 mg/dl does not apply to other types of lower-risk individuals who do not have CHD or other forms of atherosclerotic disease; in such cases, recommendations contained in the 2004 ATP III update still pertain [1].

In view of the lack of an effect of the current intensive lipid-lowering (statins as monotherapy) strategy on overall mortality, it is logical to ask whether other strategies could be more beneficial and safer. The relative safety and efficacy of other strategies such as combination treatment of statins with nicotinic acid derivatives, fibrates, and ezetimibe will need to be determined. Moreover, current therapeutic use of statins as monotherapy even in optimal doses and achieved target LDL-C reduction is still leaving many patients with mixed atherogenic dyslipidemia at high risk for coronary events. Targeting multiple lipid pathways can provide greater reductions in LDL-C as well as improvements in other lipid parameters. Combination therapy with agents with complementary mechanisms may enable more patients to be treated to recommended targets for optimal CAD risk reduction [22, 23].

Fibrates

Fibrates have been used in clinical practice for more than four decades due to their ability to substantially decrease triglyceride levels, to increase HDL-cholesterol levels and in addition to reduce LDL-C moderately but significant [9].

Due to their beneficial effects on glucose and lipid metabolism, peroxisome proliferators-activated receptors (PPARs) and alpha agonists (fibrates) are good potential candidates for reducing the risk of MI in subjects with metabolic syndrome and diabetes [24–26]. Although less clinical intervention studies have been performed with fibrates than with statins, there is evidence indicating that fibrates may reduce the risk of cardiovascular disease and particularly non-fatal MI [27–33]. Interestingly, reduction of cardiovascular disease with two of the fibric acid derivates – gemfibrozil and bezafibrate – was more pronounced in patients displaying baseline characteristics very similar to metabolic syndrome definitions [27, 28, 34].

There have been no direct head-to-head comparisons of a statin with a fibrate in any clinical endpoint trial. However, compared with statins, fibrates appear to more selectively target the therapeutic goals in obese individuals with features of insulin resistance and metabolic syndrome (i.e. with near-goal LDL-C and inappropriate HDL-C and triglyceride levels).

Gemfibrozil: Confirmed Long-Term Efficacy
The primary-prevention trial Helsinki Heart Study (HHS) showed that treatment with gemfibrozil led to a significant reduction in major cardiovascular

events [27]. Regarding secondary prevention, in the VAHIT study (Veterans Affairs High-density lipoprotein cholesterol Intervention Trial) – which included 30% of diabetic patients – gemfibrozil reduced the occurrence of major cardiovascular events by 22% [28]. Similarly, reduction of cardiovascular disease with gemfibrozil was more pronounced in patients displaying more than three of the features of metabolic syndrome [35, 36].

The 18-year results from the Helsinki Heart Study shows that patients in the original gemfibrozil group had a 23% lower risk of CHD mortality compared with the original placebo group. But those in the highest tertile of both body mass index and triglyceride level at baseline had the most dramatic risk reductions with gemfibrozil – 71% for CHD mortality and 33% for all-cause mortality [37].

These results are entirely consistent with the original positive results of HHS and are strongly supported by the findings of VA-HIT.

Fenofibrate: Disappointing Results of the FIELD

The recent Fenofibrate Intervention and Event Lowering in Diabetes (FIELD) study [38] investigated the effects of fenofibrate on cardiovascular events in type 2 diabetes patients. This was a multinational, randomized, double-blind, placebo-controlled trial in 9,795 subjects aged 50–75 years of age with type 2 diabetes who were not prescribed statins therapy at study entry. The primary endpoint was coronary events (CHD death or nonfatal myocardial infarction). The prespecified endpoint for subgroup analyses was cardiovascular events (cardiovascular death, myocardial infarction, stroke, and coronary and carotid revascularization procedures). After 5 years, fenofibrate-treated patients had a nonsignificant 11% reduction in the incidence of the primary endpoint, nonfatal myocardial infarction, or CHD death (5.2% event rate for the fenofibrate group compared with 5.9% for the placebo group; p = 0.16). Fenofibrate treatment did, however, reduce the incidence of the broader total cardiovascular events endpoint (a prespecified secondary endpoint) by 11% (p = 0.035). Fenofibrate reduced the incidence of most other prespecified endpoints of macrovascular disease, including nonfatal myocardial infarction events by 24% (p = 0.01), coronary revascularizations by 21% (p = 0.003), and all revascularizations by 20% (p = 0.001). Fenofibrate treatment had a particularly beneficial effect in patients that had no prior CHD. In this primary prevention population (78% of the total population), fenofibrate reduced the incidence of the primary endpoint (CHD events) by 25% (p = 0.014) and the incidence of total cardiovascular events by 19% (p = 0.004). In addition, fenofibrate unexpectedly showed statistically significant reductions in several endpoints, suggesting that a microvascular benefit was provided by this treatment. These included a reduction in the requirement for laser retinopathy (5.2 vs. 3.6%, for a 30% reduction; p = 0.0003) and a reduction in albuminuria (2.5% absolute reduction and 1.2% regression; p = 0.002).

The FIELD study design allowed for statins therapy or other lipid-lowering drugs to be added at any time after randomization to either the fenofibrate arm or the placebo arm. The average use of other lipid-lowering therapies (mainly statins) was 17% in the placebo patients and 8% in the fenofibrate patients (p < 0.0001). Significant differences also existed in the use of other in-treatment therapies between the two treatment arms, including angiotensin-converting enzyme (ACE) inhibitors (p = 0.003), beta blockers (p = 0.01), diuretics (p = 0.006), and coronary revascularization procedures (p = 0.003), with the greater use always occurring in placebo patients. There was a continual increase in statins use through the course of the study, and by the end of the study the statins drop-in rate was 36% in the placebo patients and 19% in the fenofibrate patients. Initiation of statins therapy and other secondary preventive therapies such as aspirin, ACE inhibitors, and beta blockers also occurred at higher rates in patients with a prior history of CHD compared with patients with no prior history of CHD. The differential use of statins and other evidence-based therapies significantly attenuated the benefits of fenofibrate therapy. Adjustment for statins use revealed a pronounced reduction of total cardiovascular events.

A second explanation for the negative outcome of FIELD related to the change in lipids with fenofibrate, which was considerably less than expected for HDL cholesterol: it was increased by just 5% (compare, for example, with 18% increasing of HDL-C by bezafibrate in the BIP trial).

Bezafibrate: Emerged Benefits in Metabolic Syndrome

Bezafibrate, in comparison with other fibrates, has a unique characteristic profile of action since it activates all three PPAR subtypes (alpha, gamma and delta) at comparable doses [39–41]. Therefore, bezafibrate operates as a pan-agonist for all three PPAR isoforms. In two old studies bezafibrate decreased the rate of progression of coronary atherosclerosis and decreased coronary event rate [29, 30]. In another large trial in 1,568 men with lower extremity arterial disease, bezafibrate reduced the severity of intermittent claudication [31]. In general, the incidence of coronary heart disease in patients on bezafibrate has tended to be lower, but this tendency did not reach statistical significance. However, bezafibrate had significantly reduced the incidence of nonfatal coronary events, particularly in those aged <65 years at entry, in whom all coronary events may also be reduced. In the Bezafibrate Infarction Prevention (BIP) study an overall trend of a 9.4% reduction of the incidence of primary end point (fatal or nonfatal myocardial infarction or sudden death) was observed. The reduction in the primary end point in 459 patients with high baseline triglycerides (USD 200 mg/dl) was significant [32].

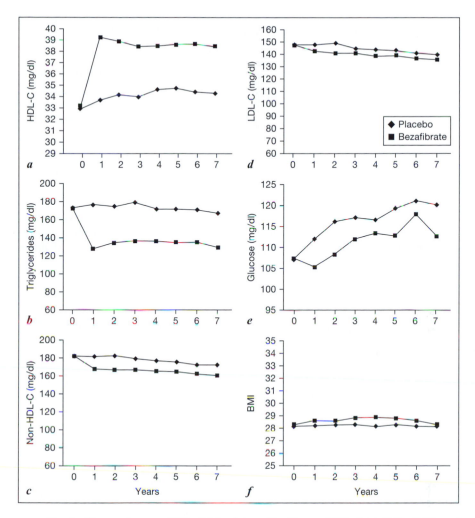

Fig. 1. Changes in mean HDL-C (*a*), triglyceride (*b*), non-HDL-C (*c*), LDL-C (*d*), and mean fasting blood glucose (*e*) levels, and body mass index (BMI) (calculated as weight in kilograms divided by the square of height in meters) (*f*) values throughout the study period (bezafibrate retard vs. placebo) following annual measurements.

Most recent extensions of the BIP trial give further support to the hypothesis that patients with insulin-resistant syndromes such as diabetes or metabolic syndrome might be the ones to derive the most benefit from therapy with fibrates [34, 42–44]. Bezafibrate can improve the metabolic profile and reduce the incidence of MI in patients with metabolic syndrome (figs 1, 2). Overall, bezafibrate treatment was associated with reduced risk of any MI and nonfatal

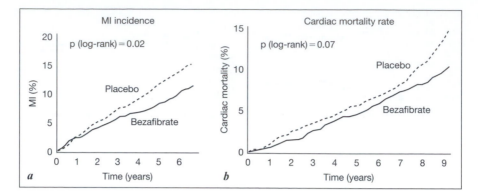

Fig. 2. Kaplan-Meier curves of the incidence of myocardial infarction (*a*) (in accordance with the time of diagnosis; mean follow-up, 6.2 years) and cardiac mortality rate (*b*) (mean follow-up, 8.1 years) for the study groups (bezafibrate retard vs. placebo). Modified from Tenenbaum et al. [34].

MI with HR (CI), respectively: 0.71 (0.54–0.95) and 0.67 (0.49–0.91). The cardiac mortality risk tended to be lower on bezafibrate (HR 0.74, CI 0.54–1.03). This trend persisted in patients with augmented features of metabolic syndrome (at least 4 risk factors for metabolic syndrome); of note, a marked reduction in cardiac mortality was observed among these patients on bezafibrate (HR 0.44, CI 0.25–0.80).

Measurements obtained during placebo treatment within the BIP trial demonstrated a natural history of progressive increasing of insulin resistance over long-term follow-up [42]. Moreover, in diabetic patients a progressive decline of pancreatic beta cell function was observed [45]. These unfavorable longitudinal changes were stopped when patients used bezafibrate [42, 45]. In addition, reduced incidence of type 2 diabetes in patients on bezafibrate has been demonstrated [43, 44]. These new data raise the intriguing possibility that bezafibrate and other fibrates may eventually prove to be clinically useful for conditions other than dyslipidemia [46].

The factor that dominates in overweight-related metabolic syndrome is the permanent elevation of plasma free fatty acids (FFA) and the predominant utilization of lipids by the muscle inducing a diminution of glucose uptake and insulin resistance. Currently, an insulin-resistant state – as the key phase of metabolic syndrome – constitutes the major risk factor for development of macrovascular complications [47–50].

On the basis of the current concept of the evolution of adipogenesis via PPAR modulation toward insulin resistance and atherothrombotic macrovascular complications (including MI), the decreasing of plasma FFA and improving of insulin sensitization by PPAR agonists seems to be a logical and valuable goal for therapy.

It is important to note that on a whole-body level, lipid and glucose metabolisms interact intimately. Briefly, PPAR alpha is activated by fibric acids (e.g. bezafibrate) and form heterodimers with the 9-cis-retinoic acid receptor (RXR). These heterodimers bind to peroxisome proliferator response elements, which are located in numerous gene promoters and increase the level of the expression of mRNAs encoded by PPAR alpha target genes. Bezafibrate reduces triglyceride plasma levels through increases in the expression of genes involved in fatty acid-beta oxidation and by a decrease in apolipoprotein C-III gene expression. Fibric acids increase HDL-C partly by increasing apolipoprotein A-I and apolipoprotein A-II gene expression. Their triglyceride-lowering and HDL-C-raising effects lead to decreased systemic availability of fatty acid, diminished fatty acid uptake by muscle with improvement of insulin sensitization and reduced plasma glucose level [51–54].

Evidence also suggests that there is a 'fibrate effect' that mediates the reduction in CHD risk beyond the favorable impact of these agents on HDL-C levels. This last notion is consistent with the pleiotropic effects of fibrates which are known to be related to their mechanisms of action [55]. Through PPAR alpha, fibrates have a significant impact on the synthesis of several apolipoproteins (apo) and enzymes of lipoprotein metabolism as well as on the expression of several genes involved in fibrinolysis and inflammation. Such changes contribute to improve the catabolism of triglyceride-rich lipoproteins, leading to a substantial increase in HDL-C levels accompanied by a shift in the size and density of LDL particles: from small, dense LDL particles to larger, more buoyant cholesteryl ester-rich LDL. These observations becomes particularly important given the dramatic increase in obesity, diabetes, and metabolic syndrome, conditions associated with low HDL and high triglyceride levels and small, dense LDL particles, the lipid profile for which fibrates would seem to be ideally suited [46].

However, different fibrates may have a somewhat different spectrum of effects. Bezafibrate as a pan-PPAR activator has clearly demonstrated beneficial pleiotropic effects related to glucose metabolism and insulin sensitivity. The recent collaborative Israeli-Japanese study had shown that bezafibrate significantly increased adiponectin levels both in humans and rodents. This effect was mediated mostly via PPAR alpha, but partially via PPAR gamma as well [56]. Bezafibrate effectively ameliorates atherogenic dyslipidemia by reducing remnants and small LDL as well as by increasing HDL particles in hypertriglyceridemic subjects [57] and induced plaque regression in thoracic and abdominal aortas [58]. Therefore, pooled together evidence suggests that gemfibrozil and bezafibrate have optimum cardiovascular benefit in metabolic syndrome and/or other appearances of insulin resistance.

Nicotinic Acid

Nicotinic acid (or niacin) has beneficial effects on all traditional blood lipid and lipoprotein fractions, particularly for increasing HDL-C and reducing lipoprotein(a). Nicotinic acid has been used for the treatment of dyslipidemia since the 1950s, but the mechanism of action has only recently been elucidated. Niacin, a vitamin of the B complex which participates in tissue respiration oxidation-reduction reactions, decreases the fractional catabolic rate of apoA-I via reduction in hepatocyte uptake [59]. Increasing apoA-I would facilitate greater RCT by making apoA-I more bioavailable to remove excess cellular cholesterol from the arterial wall macrophage. Niacin also inhibits hepatic diacylglycerol acyltransferase 2 (DGAT2) which is a key enzyme in the synthesis of triglycerides destined for VLDL [60]. Nicotinic acid additionally inhibits adipose tissue lipolysis by inhibiting hormone-sensitive triglyceride lipase [61]. It is through this combination of action that nicotinic acid exerts its changes upon lipid parameters – increased HDL, lowered LDL and triglycerides – and the clinical consequences of these effects have been positively borne out in clinical trials.

The benefits of niacin therapy upon cardiovascular events and mortality was first demonstrated in the Coronary Drug Project (CDP), a randomized, double-blind, placebo-controlled trial on 8,341 men with prior myocardial infarction that was started in 1966 [62]. Significantly fewer cardiovascular events and a mortality benefit were seen at the conclusion of the original trial after 6 years of follow-up, and these results persisted 15 years after the initiation of niacin [63]. Niacin therapy, however, is poorly tolerated by patients primarily because of skin flushing. Of subjects taking immediate-release niacin, 85% experience flushing [64]; in fact, 75% of patients in the niacin arm of the CDP dropped out of the study [65]. The flushing issue has been ameliorated by the introduction of slow-release niacins – flushing for these products is approximately 26% [64] – and premedication with aspirin. However, slow-release niacins lead to hepatotoxicity, which appear to be caused by metabolites of the nicotinamide metabolic pathway.

New prolonged-release nicotinic acid designed to produce less vasodilatory flushing than crystalline immediate-release nicotinic acid and less hepatotoxicity than previous sustained-release formulations of nicotinic acid [66]. Despite the benefit of this therapy, patient adherence is poor. Nicotinic acid has also been criticized for dysregulation of glycemic control [67]: nicotinic acid therapy, particularly in large doses, can decrease insulin sensitivity and increase plasma glucose levels [68, 69]. Probably, this effect for prolonged-release nicotinic acid is less than previously reported for crystalline nicotinic acid [70].

Bile Acid Sequestrants

There are three most popular bile acid sequestrants: cholestyramine, colesevelam, and colestipol. The principal mechanism of action of these drugs is the binding of bile acids within the intestinal lumen thereby reducing the reabsorption of bile acids and available intrahepatic cholesterol. Partial diversion of the enterohepatic circulation using bile acid sequestrants depletes the endogenous bile acid pool by approximately 40%, thus stimulating an increase in bile acid synthesis from cholesterol, which lowers LDL-C by 15–26%. The mechanism by which HDL is raised is through increased intestinal production of apoA-I [71]. The largest trial to study a bile acid sequestrant as monotherapy for hypercholesterolemia was the Lipid Research Clinics Coronary Primary Prevention Trial. This trial of 3,806 hypercholesterolemic men without CHD found a 19% reduction in the incidence of CHD in the men treated with cholestyramine [72]. Bile acid sequestrants are not absorbed by the intestine and thus have no systemic drug-drug interactions, but may interfere with the absorption of some drugs [73]. The use of bile acid sequestrants is limited by patient adherence as these drugs commonly cause gastrointestinal side effects, especially constipation, and require large and frequent dosing. The effect on HDL elevation is usually negligible. Lastly, for the dyslipidemic patient who concomitantly has high triglycerides, these drugs have no beneficial effect.

Why Ezetimibe Could Be Effective for Atherogenic Dyslipidemia?

Ezetimibe is a novel cholesterol absorption inhibitor that blocks the translocation of dietary and biliary cholesterol from the gastrointestinal lumen into the intracellular space of jejunal enterocytes [74]. Similar to the bile acid sequestrants, ezetimibe reduces intestinal cholesterol absorption by binding to the apical cholesterol export pumps ABC proteins. The ABC transporters are located in the intestinal enterocytes brush border and promote efflux of dietary cholesterol and plant sterols from enterocytes back into the intestinal lumen, thus limiting the amount of absorbed cholesterol [75]. The newly identified Niemann-Pick C1-like 1 (NPC1L1) protein is expressed at the apical membrane of enterocytes and plays a crucial role in the ezetimibe-sensitive cholesterol absorption pathway.

Experimental models suggest that ezetimibe, similar to other lipid-modifying agents, results in reduced atherosclerosis; in apoE-knockout mice, ezetimibe

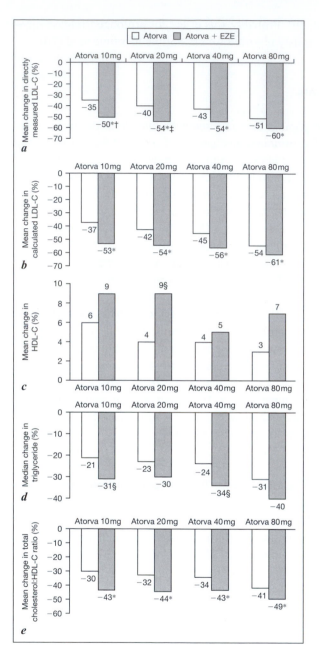

Fig. 3. Change in direct LDL-C (***a***), calculated LDL-C (***b***), HDL-C (***c***), and triglyceride (***d***) concentrations and total cholesterol:HDL-C ratio (***e***) from baseline to final assessment in patients with primary hypercholesterolemia. Atorva indicates atorvastatin; EZE = ezetimibe. $p < 0.01$ for combination therapy vs *corresponding dose of atorvastatin alone; † = atorvastatin

administration resulted in reduced carotid and aortic atherosclerotic development [76]. Ezetimibe effectively lowers circulating LDL-C levels both when administered as monotherapy and especially in combination with other hypolipidemic drugs, mostly statins [77, 78]. The coadministration of ezetimibe with a statin has yet to be proven to have a morbidity or mortality advantage over statins monotherapy and clinical trials are in development.

Meanwhile, the ENHANCE study (720 patients with familial hypercholesterolemia) showed no difference in the progression of carotid atherosclerosis between a combination of ezetimibe/simvastatin 10/80 mg vs. simvastatin 80 mg alone over a 2-year period. This was a surrogate end point that was not powered or designed to assess cardiovascular clinical event outcomes. The safety profiles were similar and there were no cases of rhabdomyolysis. Conclusions should not be made until the three large clinical outcome trials that involve more than 20,000 high-risk patients will be completed within the next 2–3 years.

Nonetheless, ezetimibe/statins combinations provide superior lipid-modifying benefits compared with any statins monotherapy in patients with atherogenic dyslipidemia typical for type 2 diabetes or metabolic syndrome [79]. Atherogenic dyslipidemia is associated with increased levels of chylomicrons and their remnants – triglyceride-rich lipoproteins (TRLs) containing 3 main components: apolipoprotein B-48 (apoB-48), triglycerides and cholesterol ester of intestinal origin. Theoretically, reduction in accessibility for one of them (specifically cholesteryl ester lessening due to ezetimibe administration) could lead to a decrease in the entire production of chylomicrons and results in a decrease of the hepatic and whole body triglycerides pool. Indeed, a number of clinical studies demonstrated that ezetimibe reduces the triglycerides level both as monotherapy and in combination with statins or fibrate (figs 3, 4) [80–83].

Overall, ezetimibe has a favorable drug-drug interaction profile, as evidenced by the lack of clinically relevant interactions between ezetimibe and a variety of drugs commonly used in patients with hypercholesterolemia. Ezetimibe does not have significant effects on plasma levels of statins, fibrates, digoxin, glipizide, warfarin and triphasic oral contraceptives. Higher ezetimibe exposures were observed in patients receiving concomitant ciclosporin, and ezetimibe caused a small but statistically significant effect on plasma levels of ciclosporin. Because treatment experience in patients receiving ciclosporin is limited, physicians are advised to exercise caution when initiating ezetimibe in the setting of ciclosporin coadministration, and to carefully monitor ciclosporin levels.

(20 mg or 40 mg) alone; ‡ = atorvastatin (40 mg) alone; § = $p < 0.05$ for combination therapy vs corresponding dose of atorvastatin alone. It should be pointed that coadministration of ezetimibe with atorvastatin provided greater reductions for triglycerides and greater increase in HDL-C (*c* and *d*) than atorvastatin alone. Modified from Ballantyne et al. [81].

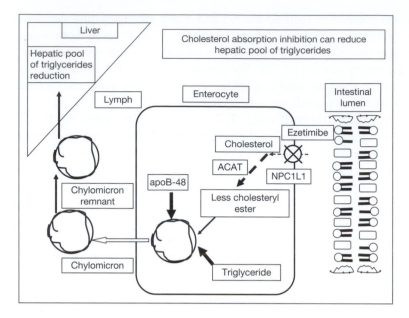

Fig. 4. Atherogenic dyslipidemia is associated with increased levels of chylomicrons and their remnants containing 3 main components: apolipoprotein B-48 (apoB-48), triglycerides and cholesterol ester of intestinal origin. Reduction in accessibility for cholesteryl ester due to ezetimibe administration could lead to decrease entire production of chylomicrons and results decreasing of hepatic triglycerides pool. ACAT = Acyl coenzyme A cholesteryl acyltransferase; NPC1L1 = Niemann-Pick C1-like 1 protein.

Cholesteryl Ester Transfer Protein Inhibition

Increasing HDL-C levels by pharmacological inhibition of the cholesteryl ester transfer protein (CETP) was until recently under intense investigation. Two small-molecule compounds, JTT-705 and torcetrapib, have been shown to effectively increase HDL-C levels in humans [84–85]. However, whether this approach will translate into a reduction in risk of atherosclerotic disease had not been clarified. Elevated HDL secondary to CETP deficiency may not be atheroprotective. An inhibition of CETP would allow the accumulation of lipid-laden HDL, but not lipid-deficient HDL. One hypothesis that could support the epidemiologic findings is that although HDL is increased, more atherogenic low-density particles could accumulate, and if HDL is already lipid-laden, there would be less lipid-deficient HDL to participate in RCT. Animal models suggest that partial inhibition of CETP results in reduced atherosclerosis. Clinical trials of CETP inhibitors in humans have resulted in impressive increases in

HDL. Torcetrapib, a small molecule inhibitor of CETP, increased HDL by 46–106% without any significant change in other lipid parameters [86]. Another small molecule inhibitor JTT-705 increased HDL by 34% with a modest 7% decrease in LDL [87]. However, the effectiveness of CETP inhibition as a strategy for antiatherosclerotic therapy has been controversial [86–91]. Specific concern about the benefits and risks of torcetrapib emerged when initial clinical trials demonstrated a dose-dependent increase in blood pressure [92]. Several potential mechanisms could explain the lack of antiatherosclerotic efficacy observed in the torcetrapib-atorvastatin group. The increase in systolic blood pressure observed in this group may have counterbalanced any benefits derived from the increases in HDL-C levels and decreases in LDL-C levels. The functionality of HDL-C produced through CETP inhibition remains uncertain. The possibility that the HDL-C produced by torcetrapib might be dysfunctional deserves careful consideration. The increase in blood pressure observed in torcetrapib-treated patients may reflect more generalized vascular toxicity, effects that could have counterbalanced any antiatherosclerotic benefits derived from an increase in HDL-C. Phase III clinical trials of this drug were recently stopped because 82 patients taking torcetrapib and atorvastatin died, compared with only 52 deaths in those on atorvastatin alone [21]. Following these results and in interests of patient safety, Pfizer stopped all torcetrapib clinical trials [93, 94].

Omega–3 Long-Chain Polyunsaturated Fatty Acids

Epidemiologic studies have reported a lower prevalence of impaired glucose tolerance and type 2 diabetes in populations consuming large amounts of the omega–3 long-chain polyunsaturated fatty acids (omega–3 LC-PUFAs) found mainly in fish [95–97]. The two marine omega–3 fatty acids eicosapentaenoic acid (EPA) and docosahexaenoic acid (DHA), prevalent in fish and fish oils, have been investigated as a strategy towards prophylaxis of atherosclerosis.

For dietetics professionals in clinical practice, appropriate dietary guidance for patients with metabolic syndrome should incorporate the recommendation to consume fatty fish, such as salmon, rainbow trout, sardines, mackerel, and herring, at least twice a week. Two to three 3-oz servings of fatty fish per week, containing at least 1 g per serving of EPA and DHA, would provide about 300–450 mg omega–3 LC-PUFAs per day. Slightly larger serving size (3.5–4 oz) of certain fatty fish, such as king, sockeye, pink, and Atlantic (farmed) salmon, consumed three times per week easily provides about 850 mg EPA and DHA per day [98, 99].

However, sources of EPA and DHA devoid of methyl-mercury (founded in many fatty fishes) are preferable, since methyl-mercury is a risk factor for cardiovascular disease.

Omega–3 fatty acids supplementation reduces plasma triacylglycerols and improves the lipoprotein profile by decreasing the fraction of atherogenic small, dense LDL and may increase HDL-C levels. However, EPA and DHA do not lower LDL-C. These effects are likely mediated through the activity of transcription factors relating to expression of genes involved in lipid oxidation and synthesis. Other pleiotrophic effects of EPA and DHA may contribute to decreasing the burden of the metabolic syndrome, such as modulating inflammation, platelet activation, endothelial function, and blood pressure [95–100]. Omega–3 fatty acids have beneficial effects in reducing remnant lipoprotein levels in persons with obesity and type 2 diabetes [101].

Recent studies using low doses of omega–3 LC-PUFAs, ranging from 1 to 2 g/day, have reported no deterioration in glucose control. The increase in glycated hemoglobin associated with the higher doses of omega–3 LC-PUFAs could be prevented by moderate exercise [101–105].

An antiarrhythmic effect of omega–3 LC-PUFAs can be demonstrated on the supraventricular and the ventricular level. More importantly, large clinical studies (The Diet and Reinfarction Trial (DART), Gruppo Italiano per lo Studio della Sopravvivenza nell'Infarto miocardico (GISSI) and Japan EPA lipid intervention study (JELIS)) showed reductions in clinical endpoints like sudden cardiac death or major adverse cardiac events [106–108].

Although differences in biological activity exist between EPA and DHA, both exert a number of positive actions against atherosclerosis and its complications. Studies comparing the effect of both major omega–3 LC-PUFAs are limited, DHA probably appears even more efficient than EPA in correcting several cardiovascular risk factors [109–111], whereas latter may be preferable for mood control (in according with number of small randomized controlled trials) [112–116]. Both EPA and DHA are equally effective in reducing serum triglycerides, but DHA and not EPA increased HDL-C and, in particular, the HDL_2 cholesterol sub-fraction. Additionally, DHA increased LDL particle size, potentially an antiatherogenic effect [109]. Neither EPA nor DHA affects total cholesterol concentrations. DHA is more effective in reducing blood pressure than EPA and these blood pressure-lowering effects correlate with improvements in endothelial relaxation and attenuated vascular constriction. DHA but not EPA also significantly decreased heart rate, suggesting that this fatty acid may be more important than EPA regarding the anti-arrhythmic effects [111].

Additional cardiovascular benefit might be realized from the synergistic effect of omega–3 LC-PUFAs with statins therapy on improved lipoprotein profiles, reduced disease progression, and lower risk of mortality [117].

Therefore, currently available evidence has shown that consumption of omega–3 LC-PUFAs in persons with type 2 diabetes and metabolic syndrome has cardioprotective effects without sizable adverse effects on glucose control. Accordingly, a number of cardiac societies have incorporated recommendations of EPA and DHA use for cardiovascular prevention into their relevant guidelines.

Combined Therapy: Approaches to Optimization of Lipid-Lowering Management

Whereas statins remain the drug of choice for patients who need to achieve the LDL-C goal, fibrates, niacin or bile acid sequestrants may represent the alternative intervention for subjects with atherogenic dyslipidemia typical for metabolic syndrome and an LDL-C already close to goal values. In addition, the concomitant use of fibrates or niacin seems to be attractive in patients whose LDL-cholesterol is controlled by statins therapy but whose HDL-cholesterol and/or triglyceride levels are still inappropriate [118–122]. This strategy will be tested in the ongoing Action to Control Cardiovascular Risk in Diabetes (ACCORD) trial [123]. Although like FIELD, fenofibrate is used in ACCORD to treat diabetes, unlike the FIELD study fenofibrate is not being used as monotherapy but only in combination with simvastatin to compare results with simvastatin therapy alone. This design should largely avoid the problem of off-trial drug use encountered in FIELD and at the same time might solidify a role for fenofibrate as a specific adjunct to statins therapy in the treatment of diabetic dyslipidemia [123].

Controlled clinical trials show similar or even greater cardiovascular benefits from statins-based therapy in patient subgroups with diabetes, impaired fasting glucose, and metabolic syndrome, compared with overall study populations [124]. Therefore, statins are the drug of first choice for aggressive lipid lowering actions and reducing risk of coronary artery disease in these patients with combined atherogenic dyslipidemia. However, current therapeutic use of statins as monotherapy is still leaving many patients with mixed atherogenic dyslipidemia at high risk for coronary events and commonly insufficient to achieve all lipid targets recommended by the current guidelines. For this reason, other approaches to treatment of combined hyperlipidemia should be considered. Because fibrates, niacin, ezetimibe and statins each regulate serum lipids by different mechanisms, combination therapy may offer particularly desirable benefits in patients with combined hyperlipidemia.

A combination statins/fibrate or statins/niacin therapy may be often necessary to control all lipid abnormalities in patients with metabolic syndrome and diabetes adequately, since fibrates and niacin provide additional important benefits, particularly on triglyceride and HDL-C levels. Thus, this combined therapy concentrates on all the components of the mixed dyslipidemia that often occurs in persons with diabetes or metabolic syndrome, and may be expected to reduce cardiovascular morbidity and mortality.

Safety concerns about some fibrates such as gemfibrozil may lead to exaggerate precautions regarding fibrate administration and therefore diminish the use of these agents. However, other fibrates (such as bezafibrate and fenofibrate) appear to be safer and better tolerated [125–131]. Additionally, bezafibrate as pan-PPAR-activator has clearly demonstrated beneficial pleiotropic effects related to glucose metabolism and insulin sensitivity. Therefore, a proper co-administration of statins with other agents – fibrates, niacin [132] or ezetimibe [133] – selected on the basis of their safety and effectiveness, could be more valuable in achieving a comprehensive lipid control as compared with statins monotherapy.

In addition, statins therapy may be needed to offset the secondary increase in levels of LDL cholesterol that frequently results from treatment with a triglyceride-lowering agent in patients with marked hypertriglyceridemia. In a number of small studies, the combination of statins and omega–3 fatty acids has been consistently shown to be an effective, safe, and well-tolerated treatment for combined dyslipidemia. Patients with recent myocardial infarction may also benefit from this combination. When considering risks and benefits of adding a second agent to statins for treatment of combined dyslipidemia, omega–3 fatty acids provide additional lipid improvements without requiring additional laboratory tests and do not increase the risk for adverse muscle or liver effects.

Because fibrates, niacin, ezetimibe, omega–3 fatty acids and statins each regulate serum lipids by different mechanisms, combination therapy may offer particularly desirable benefits in patients with combined atherogenic hyperlipidemia.

Acknowledgements

This work was supported in part by the Cardiovascular Diabetology Research Foundation (RA 58–040–684–1), Holon, Israel, and the Research Authority of Tel-Aviv University (Citernick grant 01250239).

References

1   Smith SC Jr, Allen J, Blair SN, Bonow RO, Brass LM, Fonarow GC, Grundy SM, Hiratzka L, Jones D, Krumholz HM, Mosca L, Pasternak RC, Pearson T, Pfeffer MA, Taubert KA, AHA/ACC, National Heart, Lung, and Blood Institute: AHA/ACC guidelines for secondary prevention for

patients with coronary and other atherosclerotic vascular disease: 2006 update: endorsed by the National Heart, Lung, and Blood Institute. Circulation 2006;113:2363–2372.

2 Cannon CP, Braunwald E, McCabe CH, Rader DJ, Rouleau JL, Belder R, Joyal SV, Hill KA, Pfeffer MA, Skene AM, Pravastatin or Atorvastatin Evaluation and Infection Therapy-Thrombolysis in Myocardial Infarction 22 Investigators: Intensive versus moderate lipid lowering with statins after acute coronary syndromes. N Engl J Med 2004;350:1495–1504.

3 de Lemos JA, Blazing MA, Wiviott SD, Lewis EF, Fox KA, White HD, Rouleau JL, Pedersen TR, Gardner LH, Mukherjee R, Ramsey KE, Palmisano J, Bilheimer DW, Pfeffer MA, Califf RM, Braunwald E, A to Z Investigators: Early intensive vs. a delayed conservative simvastatin strategy in patients with acute coronary syndromes: phase Z of the A to Z trial. JAMA 2004;292: 1307–1316.

4 LaRosa JC, Grundy SM, Waters DD, Shear C, Barter P, Fruchart JC, Gotto AM, Greten H, Kastelein JJ, Shepherd J, Wenger NK, Treating to New Targets (TNT) Investigators: Intensive lipid lowering with atorvastatin in patients with stable coronary disease. N Engl J Med 2005;352: 1425–1435.

5 Pedersen TR, Faergeman O, Kastelein JJ, Olsson AG, Tikkanen MJ, Holme I, Larsen ML, Bendiksen FS, Lindahl C, Szarek M, Tsai J, Incremental Decrease in End Points Through Aggressive Lipid Lowering (IDEAL) Study Group: High-dose atorvastatin vs. usual-dose simvas-tatin for secondary prevention after myocardial infarction: the IDEAL study: a randomized con-trolled trial. JAMA 2005;294:2437–2445.

6 Fisman EZ, Adler Y, Tenenbaum A: Statins research unfinished saga: desirability versus feasibil-ity. Cardiovasc Diabetol 2005;4:8.

7 Christopher CP: The IDEAL cholesterol: lower is better. JAMA 2005;294:2492249–2492254.

8 Pitt B: Low-density lipoprotein cholesterol in patients with stable coronary heart disease–is it time to shift our goals? N Engl J Med 2005;352:1483–1484.

9 Tenenbaum A, Fisman EZ: Which is the best lipid-modifying strategy in metabolic syndrome and diabetes: fibrates, statins or both? Cardiovasc Diabetol 2004;3:10.

10 Cannon CP, Steinberg BA, Murphy SA, Mega JL, Braunwald E: Meta-analysis of cardiovascular outcomes trials comparing intensive versus moderate statin therapy. J Am Coll Cardiol 2006;48:438–445.

11 Begg CB: The role of meta-analysis in monitoring clinical trials. Stat Med 1996;15:1299–1306.

12 Ravnskov U, Rosch PJ, Sutter MC: Should we lower cholesterol as much as possible? BMJ 2006;332:1330–1332.

13 Muldoon MF, Ryan CM, Sereika SM, Flory JD, Manuck SB: Randomized trial of the effects of sim-vastatin on cognitive functioning in hypercholesterolemic adults. Am J Med 2004;117: 823–829.

14 Bernick C, Katz R, Smith NL, Rapp S, Bhadelia R, Carlson M, Kuller L, Cardiovascular Health Study Collaborative Research Group: Statins and cognitive function in the elderly: the Cardiovascular Health Study. Neurology 2005;65:1388–1394.

15 Law M, Rudnick AR: Statin safety: a systematic review. Am J Cardiol 2006;97:52C–60C.

16 Golomb BA: Implications of statin adverse effects in the elderly. Expert Opin Drug Saf 2005;4: 389–397.

17 King DS, Wilburn AJ, Wofford MR, Harrell TK, Lindley BJ, Jones DW: Cognitive impairment associated with atorvastatin and simvastatin. Pharmacotherapy 2003;23:1663–1667.

18 Wagstaff LR, Mitton MW, Arvik BM, Doraiswamy PM: Statin-associated memory loss: analysis of 60 case reports and review of the literature. Pharmacotherapy 2003;23:871–880.

19 Gaist D, Jeppesen U, Andersen M, Garcia Rodriguez LA, Hallas J, Sindrup SH: Statins and risk of polyneuropathy: a case-control study. Neurology 2002;58:1333–1337.

20 Rizvi K, Hampson JP, Harvey JN: Do lipid-lowering drugs cause erectile dysfunction? A system-atic review. Fam Pract 2002;19:95–98.

21 Garg A, Simha V: Update on dyslipidemia. J Clin Endocrinol Metab 2007;92:1581–1589.

22 Ballantyne CM: Rationale for targeting multiple lipid pathways for optimal cardiovascular risk reduction. Am J Cardiol 2005;96:14K–19K.

23 Tenenbaum A, Fisman EZ, Motro M, Adler Y: Atherogenic dyslipidemia in metabolic syndrome and type 2 diabetes: therapeutic options beyond statins. Cardiovasc Diabetol 2006;5:20.

Management of Combined Dyslipidemia

24 Sacks FM, for the Expert Group on HDL Cholesterol: The role of high-density lipoprotein [HDL] cholesterol in the prevention and treatment of coronary heart disease: Expert Group recommendations. Am J Cardiol 2002;90:139–143.

25 Fruchart JC: Peroxisome proliferator-activated receptor-alpha activation and high-density lipoprotein metabolism. Am J Cardiol 2001;88:24N–29N.

26 Verges B: Clinical interest of PPARs ligands. Diabetes Metab 2004;30:7–12.

27 Frick MH, Elo O, Haapa K, Heinonen OP, Heinsalmi P, Helo P, Huttunen JK, Kaitaniemi P, Koskinen P, Manninen V: Helsinki Heart Study: primary-prevention trial with gemfibrozil in middle-aged men with dyslipidemia. Safety of treatment, changes in risk factors, and incidence of coronary heart disease. N Engl J Med 1987;317:1237–1245.

28 Rubins HB, Robins SJ, Collins D, Fye CL, Anderson JW, Elam MB, Faas FH, Linares E, Schaefer EJ, Schectman G, Wilt TJ, Wittes J: Gemfibrozil for the secondary prevention of coronary heart disease in men with low levels of high-density lipoprotein cholesterol. Veterans Affairs High-Density Lipoprotein Cholesterol Intervention Trial Study Group. N Engl J Med 1999;341: 410–418.

29 Ericsson CG, Nilsson J, Grip L, Svane B, Hamsten A: Effect of bezafibrate treatment over five years on coronary plaques causing 20% to 50% diameter narrowing. The Bezafibrate Coronary Atherosclerosis Intervention Trial (BECAIT). Am J Cardiol 1997;8:1125–1129.

30 Elkeles RS, Diamond JR, Poulter C, Dhanjil S, Nicolaides AN, Mahmood S, Richmond W, Mather H, Sharp P, Feher MD: Cardiovascular outcomes in type 2 diabetes. A double-blind placebo-controlled study of bezafibrate: the St. Mary's, Ealing, Northwick Park Diabetes Cardiovascular Disease Prevention (SENDCAP) Study. Diabetes Care 1998;21:641–648.

31 Meade T, Zuhrie R, Cook C, Cooper J: Bezafibrate in men with lower extremity arterial disease: randomised controlled trial. BMJ 2002;325:1139.

32 Secondary prevention by raising HDL cholesterol and reducing triglycerides in patients with coronary artery disease: the Bezafibrate Infarction Prevention (BIP) study. Circulation 2000;102: 21–27.

33 Diabetes Atherosclerosis Intervention Study Investigators: Effect of fenofibrate on progression of coronary-artery disease in type 2 diabetes: the diabetes atherosclerosis intervention study, a randomised study. Lancet 2001;357:905–910.

34 Tenenbaum A, Motro M, Fisman EZ, Tanne D, Boyko V, Behar S: Bezafibrate for the secondary prevention of myocardial infarction in patients with metabolic syndrome. Arch Intern Med 2005;165:1154–1160.

35 Manninen V, Tenkanen L, Koskinen P, Huttunen JK, Manttari M, Heinonen OP, Frick MH: Joint effects of serum triglyceride and LDL cholesterol and HDL cholesterol concentrations on coronary heart disease risk in the Helsinki Heart Study: implications for treatment. Circulation 1992;85:37–45.

36 Rubins HB, Robins SJ, Collins D, Nelson DB, Elam MB, Schaefer EJ, Faas FH, Anderson JW: Diabetes, plasma insulin, and cardiovascular disease: subgroup analysis from the Department of Veterans Affairs high-density lipoprotein intervention trial (VA-HIT). Arch Intern Med 2002;162:2597–2604.

37 Tenkanen L, Manttari M, Kovanen P, et al: Gemfibrozil in the treatment of dyslipidemia: an 18-year mortality follow-up of the Helsinki Heart Study. Arch Intern Med 2006;166:743–748.

38 Keech A, Simes RJ, Barter P, Best J, Scott R, Taskinen MR, Forder P, Pillai A, Davis T, Glasziou P, Drury P, Kesaniemi YA, Sullivan D, Hunt D, Colman P, d'Emden M, Whiting M, Ehnholm C, Laakso M, FIELD Study Investigators: Effects of long-term fenofibrate therapy on cardiovascular events in 9795 people with type 2 diabetes mellitus (the FIELD study): randomised controlled trial. Lancet 2005;366:1849–1861.

39 Willson TM, Brown PJ, Sternbach DD, Henke BR: The PPARs: from orphan receptors to drug discovery. J Med Chem 2000;43:527–550.

40 Berger J, Moller DE: The mechanisms of action of PPARs. Annu Rev Med 2002;53:409–435.

41 Tenenbaum A, Motro M, Fisman EZ: Dual and pan-peroxisome proliferator-activated receptors (PPAR) co-agonism: the bezafibrate lessons. Cardiovasc Diabetol 2005;4:14.

42   Tenenbaum A, Fisman EZ, Boyko V, Benderly M, Tanne D, Haim M, Matas Z, Motro M, Behar S: Attenuation of progression of insulin resistance in patients with coronary artery disease by bezafibrate. Arch Intern Med 2006;166:737–741.

43   Tenenbaum A, Motro M, Fisman EZ, Schwammenthal E, Adler Y, Goldenberg I, Leor J, Boyko V, Mandelzweig L, Behar S: Peroxisome proliferator-activated receptors ligand bezafibrate for prevention of type 2 diabetes mellitus in patients with coronary artery disease. Circulation 2004;109:2197–2202.

44   Tenenbaum A, Motro M, Fisman EZ, Adler Y, Shemesh J, Tanne D, Leor J, Boyko V, Schwammenthal E, Behar S: Effect of bezafibrate on incidence of type 2 diabetes mellitus in obese patients. Eur Heart J 2005;26:2032–2038.

45   Tenenbaum H, Behar S, Boyko V, Adler Y, Fisman EZ, Tanne D, Lapidot M, Schwammenthal E, Feinberg M, Matas Z, Motro M, Tenenbaum A: Long-term effect of bezafibrate on pancreatic beta-cell function and insulin resistance in patients with diabetes. Atherosclerosis 2006;[Epub ahead of print].

46   Bloomfield HE: The role of fibrates in a statin world. Arch Intern Med 2006;166:715–716.

47   Groop LC: Insulin resistance: the fundamental trigger of type 2 diabetes. Diabetes Obes Metab 1999;(suppl 1):S1–S7.

48   Tenenbaum A, Fisman EZ, Motro M: Metabolic syndrome and type 2 diabetes mellitus: focus on peroxisome proliferator activated receptors (PPAR). Cardiovasc Diabetol 2003;2:4.

49   Lakka HM, Laaksonen DE, Lakka TA, Niskanen LK, Kumpusalo E, Tuomilehto J, Salonen JT: The metabolic syndrome and total and cardiovascular disease mortality in middle-aged men. JAMA 2002;288:2709–2716.

50   Fruchart JC, Staels B, Duriez P: The role of fibric acids in atherosclerosis. Curr Atheroscler Rep 2001;3:83–92.

51   Rovellini A, Sommariva D, Branchi A, Maraffi F, Montalto C, Gandini R, Fasoli A: Effects of slow release bezafibrate on the lipid pattern and on blood glucose of type 2 diabetic patients with hyperlipidaemia. Pharmacol Res 1992;25:237–245.

52   Taniguchi A, Fukushima M, Sakai M, Tokuyama K, Nagata I, Fukunaga A, Kishimoto H, Doi K, Yamashita Y, Matsuura T, Kitatani N, Okumura T, Nagasaka S, Nakaishi S, Nakai Y: Effects of bezafibrate on insulin sensitivity and insulin secretion in non-obese Japanese type 2 diabetic patients. Metabolism 2001;50:477–480.

53   Jonkers IJ, Mohrschladt MF, Westendorp RG, van der Laarse A, Smelt AH: Severe hypertriglyceridemia with insulin resistance is associated with systemic inflammation: reversal with bezafibrate therapy in a randomized controlled trial. Am J Med 2002;112:275–280.

54   Jones IR, Swai A, Taylor R, Miller M, Laker MF, Alberti KG: Lowering of plasma glucose concentrations with bezafibrate in patients with moderately controlled NIDDM. Diabetes Care 1990;13:855–863.

55   Despres JP, Lemieux I, Robins SJ: Role of fibric Acid derivatives in the management of risk factors for coronary heart disease. Drugs 2004;64:2177–2198.

56   Hiuge A, Tenenbaum A, Maeda N, Benderly M, Kumada M, Fisman EZ, Tanne D, Matas Z, Hibuse T, Fujita K, Nishizawa H, Adler Y, Motro M, Kihara S, Shimomura I, Behar S, Funahashi T: Effects of peroxisome proliferator-activated receptor ligands, bezafibrate and fenofibrate, on adiponectin level. Arterioscler Thromb Vasc Biol 2007;27:635–641.

57   Ikewaki K, Noma K, Tohyama J, Kido T, Mochizuki S: Effects of bezafibrate on lipoprotein subclasses and inflammatory markers in patients with hypertriglyceridemia–a nuclear magnetic resonance study. Int J Cardiol 2005;101:441–447.

58   Ayaori M, Momiyama Y, Fayad ZA, Yonemura A, Ohmori R, Kihara T, Tanaka N, Nakaya K, Ogura M, Sawada S, Taniguchi H, Kusuhara M, Nagata M, Nakamura H, Ohsuzu F: Effect of bezafibrate therapy on atherosclerotic aortic plaques detected by MRI in dyslipidemic patients with hypertriglyceridemia. Atherosclerosis 2006;[Epub ahead of print].

59   Jin FY, Kamanna VS, Kashyap ML: Niacin decreases removal of high-density lipoprotein apolipoprotein A-I but not cholesterol ester by Hep G2 cells: implication for reverse cholesterol transport. Arterioscler Thromb Vasc Biol 1997;17:2020–2028.

60   Ganji SH, Tavintharan S, Zhu D, Xing Y, Kamanna VS, Kashyap ML: Niacin noncompetitively inhibits DGAT2 but not DGAT1 activity in HepG2 cells. J Lipid Res 2004;45:1835–1845.

---

61 Tunaru S, Kero J, Schaub A, Wufka C, Blaukat A, Pfeffer K, Offermanns S: PUMA-G and HM74 are receptors for nicotinic acid and mediate its anti-lipolytic effect. Nat Med 2003;9: 352–355.

62 The Coronary Drug Project: Design, methods, and baseline results. The Coronary Drug Project Research Group. Circulation 1973;47:1–50.

63 Canner PL, Furberg CD, McGovern ME: Benefits of niacin in patients with versus without the metabolic syndrome and healed myocardial infarction (from the Coronary Drug Project). Am J Cardiol 2006;97:477–479.

64 Birjmohun RS, Hutten BA, Kastelein JJ, Stroes ES: Efficacy and safety of high-density lipoprotein cholesterol-increasing compounds: a meta-analysis of randomized controlled trials. J Am Coll Cardiol 2005;45:185–197.

65 Choi BG, Vilahur G, Yadegar D, Viles-Gonzalez JF, Badimon JJ: The role of high-density lipoprotein cholesterol in the prevention and possible treatment of cardiovascular diseases. Curr Mol Med 2006;6:571–587.

66 McCormack PL, Keating GM: Prolonged-release nicotinic acid: a review of its use in the treatment of dyslipidaemia. Drugs 2005;65:2719–2740.

67 Garg A, Grundy SM: Nicotinic acid as therapy for dyslipidemia in non-insulin-dependent diabetes mellitus. JAMA 1990;264:723–726.

68 Kelly JJ, Lawson JA, Campbell LV, Storlien LH, Jenkins AB, Whitworth JA, O'Sullivan AJ: Effects of nicotinic acid on insulin sensitivity and blood pressure in healthy subjects. J Hum Hypertens 2000;14:567–572.

69 Poynten AM, Gan SK, Kriketos AD, O'Sullivan A, Kelly JJ, Ellis BA, Chisholm DJ, Campbell LV: Nicotinic acid-induced insulin resistance is related to increased circulating fatty acids and fat oxidation but not muscle lipid content. Metabolism 2003;52:699–704.

70 Vega GL, Cater NB, Meguro S, Grundy SM: Influence of extended-release nicotinic acid on non-esterified fatty acid flux in the metabolic syndrome with atherogenic dyslipidemia. Am J Cardiol 2005;95:1309–1313.

71 Shepherd J, Packard CJ, Morgan HG, Third JL, Stewart JM, Lawrie TD: The effects of cholestyramine on high density lipoprotein metabolism. Atherosclerosis 1979;33:433–444.

72 The Lipid Research Clinics Coronary Primary Prevention Trial results. II. The relationship of reduction in incidence of coronary heart disease to cholesterol lowering. JAMA 1984;251: 365–374.

73 Insull W Jr: Clinical utility of bile acid sequestrants in the treatment of dyslipidemia: a scientific review. South Med J 2006;99:257–273.

74 Toth PP, Davidson MH: Cholesterol absorption blockade with ezetimibe. Curr Drug Targets Cardiovasc Haematol Disord 2005;5:455–462.

75 Sudhop T, Lutjohann D, Kodal A, Igel M, Tribble DL, Shah S, Perevozskaya I, von Bergmann K: Inhibition of intestinal cholesterol absorption by ezetimibe in humans. Circulation 2002;106:1943–1948.

76 Davis HR Jr, Compton DS, Hoos L, Tetzloff G: Ezetimibe, a potent cholesterol absorption inhibitor, inhibits the development of atherosclerosis in ApoE knockout mice. Arterioscler Thromb Vasc Biol 2001;21:2032–2038.

77 A. Yatskar L, Fisher EA, Schwartzbard A: Ezetimibe: rationale and role in the management of hypercholesterolemia. Clin Cardiol 2006;29:52–55.

78 B. Goldberg AC, Sapre A, Liu J, Capece R, Mitchel YB: Ezetimibe Study Group: Efficacy and safety of ezetimibe coadministered with simvastatin in patients with primary hypercholesterolemia: a randomized, double-blind, placebo-controlled trial. Mayo Clin Proc 2004;79: 620–629.

79 Goldberg RB, Guyton JR, Mazzone T, Weinstock RS, Polis A, Edwards P, Tomassini JE, Tershakovec AM: Ezetimibe/simvastatin vs. atorvastatin in patients with type 2 diabetes mellitus and hypercholesterolemia: the VYTAL study. Mayo Clin Proc 2006;81:1579–1588.

80 Dujovne CA, Ettinger MP, McNeer JF, Lipka LJ, LeBeaut AP, Suresh R, Yang B, Veltri EP, Ezetimibe Study Group: Efficacy and safety of a potent new selective cholesterol absorption inhibitor, ezetimibe, in patients with primary hypercholesterolemia. Am J Cardiol 2002;90:1092–1097.

81 Ballantyne CM, Houri J, Notarbartolo A, Melani L, Lipka LJ, Suresh R, Sun S, LeBeaut AP, Sager PT, Veltri EP, Ezetimibe Study Group: Effect of ezetimibe coadministered with atorvastatin

in 628 patients with primary hypercholesterolemia: a prospective, randomized, double-blind trial. Circulation 2003;107:2409–2415.

82 Ballantyne CM, Weiss R, Moccetti T, Vogt A, Eber B, Sosef F, Duffield E, EXPLORER Study Investigators: Efficacy and safety of rosuvastatin 40 mg alone or in combination with ezetimibe in patients at high risk of cardiovascular disease (results from the EXPLORER study). Am J Cardiol 2007;99:673–680.

83 Farnier M, Roth E, Gil-Extremera B, Mendez GF, Macdonell G, Hamlin C, Perevozskaya I, Davies MJ, Kush D, Mitchel YB, Ezetimibe/Simvastatin + Fenofibrate Study Group: Efficacy and safety of the coadministration of ezetimibe/simvastatin with fenofibrate in patients with mixed hyperlipidemia. Am Heart J 2007;153:335.e1–335.e8.

84 van der Steeg WA, El-Harchaoui K, Kuivenhoven JA, Kastelein JJ: Increasing high-density lipoprotein cholesterol through cholesteryl ester transfer protein inhibition: a next step in the fight against cardiovascular disease? Curr Drug Targets Cardiovasc Haematol Disord 2005;5:481–488.

85 Schaefer EJ, Asztalos BF: Cholesteryl ester transfer protein inhibition, high-density lipoprotein metabolism and heart disease risk reduction. Curr Opin Lipidol 2006;17:394–398.

86 Brousseau ME, Schaefer EJ, Wolfe ML, Bloedon LT, Digenio AG, Clark RW, Mancuso JP, Rader DJ: Effects of an inhibitor of cholesteryl ester transfer protein on HDL cholesterol. N Engl J Med 2004;350:1505–1515.

87 de Grooth GJ, Kuivenhoven JA, Stalenhoef AF, de Graaf J, Zwinderman AH, Posma JL, van Tol A, Kastelein JJ: Efficacy and safety of a novel cholesteryl ester transfer protein inhibitor, JTT-705, in humans: a randomized phase II dose-response study. Circulation 2002;105:2159–2165.

88 Tall AR, Yvan-Charvet L, Wang N: The failure of torcetrapib: was it the molecule or the mechanism? Arterioscler Thromb Vasc Biol 2007;27:257–260.

89 Hirano K, Yamashita S, Nakajima N, et al: Genetic cholesteryl ester transfer protein deficiency is extremely frequent in the Omagari area of Japan: marked hyperalphalipoproteinemia caused by CETP gene mutation is not associated with longevity. Arterioscler Thromb Vasc Biol 1997;17: 1053–1059.

90 Morton RE, Greene DJ: Partial suppression of CETP activity beneficially modifies the lipid transfer profile of plasma. Atherosclerosis: in press.

91 Nissen SE, Tardif JC, Nicholls SJ, Revkin JH, Shear CL, Duggan WT, Ruzyllo W, Bachinsky WB, Lasala GP, Tuzcu EM, ILLUSTRATE Investigators: Effect of torcetrapib on the progression of coronary atherosclerosis. N Engl J Med 2007;356:1304–1316.

92 McKenney JM, Davidson MH, Shear CL, Revkin JH: Efficacy and safety of torcetrapib, a novel cholesteryl ester transfer protein inhibitor, in individuals with below-average high-density lipoprotein cholesterol levels on a background of atorvastatin. J Am Coll Cardiol 2006;48: 1782–1790.

93 In interests of patient safety, Pfizer stops all torcetrapib clinical trials; company has notified FDA and is in the process of notifying all clinical investigators and other regulatory authorities. Pfizer news release, December 2, 2006. (Accessed May 15, 2007, at http://www.pfizer.ca/english/newsroom/press%20releases/default.asp?s = 1&year = 2006&releaseID = 214)

94 Tanne JH: Pfizer stops clinical trials of heart drug. BMJ 2006;333:1237.

95 Siscovick DS, Raghunathan T, King I, Weinmann S, Bovbjerg VE, Kushi L, Cobb LA, Copass MK, Psaty BM, Lemaitre R, Retzlaff B, Knopp RH: Dietary intake of long-chain n-3 polyunsaturated fatty acids and the risk of primary cardiac arrest. Am J Clin Nutr 2000;71(suppl 1): S208–S212.

96 Weisman D, Motro M, Schwammenthal E, Fisman EZ, Tenenbaum A, Tanne D, Adler Y: Efficacy of omega-3 fatty acid supplementation in primary and secondary prevention of coronary heart disease. Isr Med Assoc J 2004;6:227–232.

97 Hu FB, Cho E, Rexrode KM, Albert CM, Manson JE: Fish and long-chain ω-3 fatty acid intake and risk of coronary heart disease and total mortality in diabetic women. Circulation 2003;107: 1852–1857.

98 American Diabetes Association: Evidence-based nutrition principles and recommendations for the treatment and prevention of diabetes and related complications. Diabetes Care 2002;25(suppl 1): S50–S60.

99 AHA Nutrition Committee, Kris-Etherton P, Harris WS, Appel LJ: Fish consumption, fish oil, omega-3 fatty acids and cardiovascular disease. Circulation 2002;106:2747–2757.

100   Chan DC, Watts GF, Mori TA, Barrett PH, Redgrave TG, Beilin LJ: Randomized controlled trial of the effect of n–3 fatty acid supplementation on the metabolism of apolipoprotein B-100 and chylomicron remnants in men with visceral obesity. Am J Clin Nutr 2003;77:300–307.

101   Sirtori CR, Crepaldi G, Manzato E, Mancini M, Rivellese A, Paoliett R, Pazzucconi F, Pamparana F, Stragliotto E: One-year treatment with ethyl esters of n–3 fatty acids in patients with hypertriglyceridemia and glucose intolerance, reduced triglyceridemia, total cholesterol and increased HDL-C without glycemic alteration. Atherosclerosis 1998;137:419–427.

102   Luo J, Rizkalla SW, Vidal H, Oppert JM, Colas C, Boussairi A, Guerre-Millo M, Chapuis AS, Chevalier A, Durand G, Slama G: Moderate intake of n-3 fatty acids for 2 months has no detrimental effect on glucose metabolism and could ameliorate the lipid profile in type 2 diabetic men: results of a controlled study. Diabetes Care 1998;21:717–724.

103   Dunstan DW, Mori TA, Puddey IB, Beilin LJ, Burke V, Morton AR, Stanton KG: The independent and combined effects of aerobic exercise and dietary fish intake on serum lipids and glycemic control in NIDDM: a randomized controlled study. Diabetes Care 1997;20:913–921.

104   Friedberg CE, Janssen MJ, Heine RJ, Grobbee DE: Fish oil and glycemic control in diabetes: a meta-analysis. Diabetes Care 1998;21:494–500.

105   Montori VM, Farmer A, Wollan PC, Dinneen SF: Fish oil supplementation in type 2 diabetes: a quantitative systematic review. Diabetes Care 2000;23:1407–1415.

106   Hooper L, Thompson RL, Harrison RA, et al: Risks and benefits of omega 3 fats for mortality, cardiovascular disease, and cancer: systematic review. Br Med J 2006;332:752–760.

107   von Schacky C: Omega–3 fatty acids and cardiovascular disease. Curr Opin Clin Nutr Metab Care 2007;10:129–135.

108   Yokoyama M, Origasa H, Matsuzaki M, Matsuzawa Y, Saito Y, Ishikawa Y, Oikawa S, Sasaki J, Hishida H, Itakura H, Kita T, Kitabatake A, Nakaya N, Sakata T, Shimada K, Shirato K, Japan EPA lipid intervention study (JELIS) Investigators: Effects of eicosapentaenoic acid on major coronary events in hypercholesterolaemic patients (JELIS): a randomised open-label, blinded endpoint analysis. Lancet 2007;369:1090–1098.

109   Woodman RJ, Mori TA, Burke V, Puddey IB, Watts GF, Best JD, Beilin LJ: Docosahexaenoic acid but not eicosapentaenoic acid increases LDL particle size in treated hypertensive type 2 diabetic patients. Diabetes Care 2003;26:253.

110   Morris MC, Sacks F, Rosner B: Does fish oil lower blood pressure: a meta-analysis of controlled trials. Circulation 1993;88:523–533.

111   Mori TA, Bao DQ, Burke V, et al: Docosahexaenoic acid but not eicosapentaenoic acid lowers ambulatory blood pressure and heart rate in humans. Hypertension 1999;34:253–260.

112   Freeman MP, Hibbeln JR, Wisner KL, Davis JM, Mischoulon D, Peet M, Keck PE Jr, Marangell LB, Richardson AJ, Lake J, Stoll AL: Omega–3 fatty acids: evidence basis for treatment and future research in psychiatry. J Clin Psychiatry 2006;67:1954–1967.

113   Pouwer F, Nijpels G, Beekman AT, Dekker JM, van Dam RM, Heine RJ, Snoek FJ: Fat food for a bad mood: could we treat and prevent depression in type 2 diabetes by means of omega-3 polyunsaturated fatty acids? A review of the evidence. Diabet Med 2005;22:1465–1475.

114   Stoll AL, Severus WE, Freeman MP, Rueter S, Zboyan HA, Diamond E: Omega-3 fatty acids in bipolar disorder: a preliminary double blind, placebo-controlled trial. Arch General Psychiatry 1999;56:407–412.

115   Peet M, Horrobin DF: A dose-ranging study of the effects of ethyl-eicosapentaenoate in patients with ongoing depression despite apparently adequate treatment with standard drugs. Arch Gen Psychiatry 2002;59:913–919.

116   Nemets B, Stahl Z, Belmaker RH: Addition of omega-3 fatty acid to maintenance medication treatment for recurrent unipolar depressive disorder. Am J Psychiatry 2002;159:477–479.

117   Nambi V, Ballantyne CM: Combination therapy with statins and omega-3 fatty acids. Am J Cardiol 2006;98:34i–38i.

118   Robins SJ: Cardiovascular disease with diabetes or the metabolic syndrome: should statins or fibrates be first line lipid therapy? Curr Opin Lipidol 2003;14:575–583.

119   Tenenbaum A, Motro M, Schwammenthal E, Fisman EZ: Macrovascular complications of metabolic syndrome: an early intervention is imperative. Int J Cardiol 2004;97:167–172.

120 Fazio S, Linton MF: The role of fibrates in managing hyperlipidemia: mechanisms of action and clinical efficacy. Curr Atheroscler Rep 2004;6:148–157.

121 Role of fibrates in reducing coronary risk: a UK Consensus. Curr Med Res Opin 2004;20: 241–247.

122 Tenenbaum A, Fisman EZ, Motro M: Bezafibrate and simvastatin: different beneficial effects for different therapeutic aims. J Clin Endocrinol Metab 2004;89:1978.

123 Robins SJ, Bloomfield HE: Fibric acid derivatives in cardiovascular disease prevention: results from the large clinical trials. Curr Opin Lipidol 2006;17:431–439.

124 Verges B: Role for fibrate therapy in diabetes: evidence before FIELD. Curr Opin Lipidol 2005;16:648–651.

125 Jokubaitis LA: Fluvastatin in combination with other lipid-lowering agents. Br J Clin Pract Suppl 1996;77A:28–32.

126 Gavish D, Leibovitz E, Shapira I, Rubinstein A: Bezafibrate and simvastatin combination therapy for diabetic dyslipidaemia: efficacy and safety. J Intern Med 2000;247:563–569.

127 Kyrklund C, Backman JT, Kivisto KT, Neuvonen M, Laitila J, Neuvonen PJ: Plasma concentrations of active lovastatin acid are markedly increased by gemfibrozil but not by bezafibrate. Clin Pharmacol Ther 2001;69:340–345.

128 Beggs PW, Clark DW, Williams SM, Coulter DM: A comparison of the use, effectiveness and safety of bezafibrate, gemfibrozil and simvastatin in normal clinical practice using the New Zealand Intensive Medicines Monitoring Programme (IMMP). Br J Clin Pharmacol 1999;47:99–104.

129 Farnier M, Salko T, Isaacsohn JL, Troendle AJ, Dejager S, Gonasun L: Effects of baseline level of triglycerides on changes in lipid levels from combined fluvastatin + fibrate (bezafibrate, fenofibrate, or gemfibrozil). Am J Cardiol 2003;92:794–797.

130 Farnier M: Combination therapy with an HMG-CoA reductase inhibitor and a fibric acid derivative: a critical review of potential benefits and drawbacks. Am J Cardiovasc Drugs 2003;3:169–178.

131 Shek A, Ferrill MJ: Statin-fibrate combination therapy. Ann Pharmacother 2001;35:908–917.

132 Canner PL, Berge KG, Wenger NK, Stamler J, Friedman L, Prineas RJ, Friedewald W: Fifteen year mortality in Coronary Drug Project patients: long-term benefit with niacin. J Am Coll Cardiol 1986;8:1245–1255.

133 Toth PP, Davidson MH: Simvastatin plus ezetimibe: combination therapy for the management of dyslipidaemia. Expert Opin Pharmacother 2005;6:131–139.

Prof. Alexander Tenenbaum, MD, PhD
Cardiac Rehabilitation Institute, Sheba Medical Center, Tel-Aviv University
Tel-Hashomer 52621 (Israel)
Tel. +972 3 530 2361, Fax +972 3 530 5905, E-Mail altenen@post.tau.ac.il

Fisman EZ, Tenenbaum A (eds): Cardiovascular Diabetology: Clinical, Metabolic and Inflammatory Facets. Adv Cardiol. Basel, Karger, 2008, vol 45, pp 154–170

....

Non-Insulin Antidiabetic Therapy in Cardiac Patients: Current Problems and Future Prospects

Enrique Z. Fisman[a]   *Michael Motro*[b]   *Alexander Tenenbaum*[a,b]

[a]Cardiovascular Diabetology Research Foundation, Holon, [b]Cardiac Rehabilitation Institute, the Chaim Sheba Medical Center, Tel-Hashomer, affiliated to the Sackler Faculty of Medicine, Tel-Aviv University, Tel-Aviv, Israel

Abstract

Five types of oral antihyperglycemic drugs are currently approved for the treatment of diabetes: biguanides, sulfonylureas, meglitinides, glitazones and alpha-glucosidase inhibitors. We briefly review the cardiovascular effects of the most commonly used antidiabetic drugs in these groups in an attempt to improve knowledge and awareness regarding their influences and potential risks when treating patients with coronary artery disease (CAD). Regarding biguanides, gastrointestinal disturbances such as diarrhea are frequent, and the intestinal absorption of group B vitamins and folate is impaired during chronic therapy. This deficiency may lead to increased plasma homocysteine levels which, in turn, accelerate the progression of vascular disease due to adverse effects on platelets, clotting factors, and endothelium. The existence of a graded association between homocysteine levels and overall mortality in patients with CAD is well established. In addition, metformin may lead to lethal lactic acidosis, especially in patients with clinical conditions that predispose to this complication, such as heart failure or recent myocardial infarction. Sulfonylureas avoid ischemic preconditioning. During myocardial ischemia, they may prevent opening of the ATP-dependent potassium channels, impeding the necessary hyperpolarization that protects the cell by blocking calcium influx. Meglitinides may exert similar effects due to their analogous mechanism of action. During treatment with glitazones, edema has been reported in 5% of patients, and these drugs are contraindicated in diabetics with NYHA class III or IV cardiac status. The long-term effects of alpha-glucosidase inhibitors on morbidity and mortality rates and on diabetic micro- and macrovascular complications is still unknown. Combined sulfonylurea/metformin therapy reveals additive effects on mortality. Four points should be mentioned: (1) the five oral antidiabetic drug groups present proven or potential cardiac hazards; (2) these hazards are not mere 'side effects' but are deeply rooted in the drugs' mechanisms of action; (3) current data indicate that combined glibenclamide/metformin therapy seems to present a special risk and should be avoided in the long-term management of type 2 diabetics with proven CAD, and (4) customized antihyperglycemic pharmacological approaches should be investigated for the optimal treatment of diabetic patients with heart disease. New possibilities are represented by incretin mimetic compounds, dipeptidyl peptidase (DPP)-4 inhibitors, inhaled insulin and eventually oral insulin.

Introduction

Diabetes mellitus threatens to become a global health crisis, and treating diabetes and its complications is going to dominate future health care expenditure. Type 2 diabetes accounts for about 90% of the total diabetic population, and coronary artery disease (CAD) is the most common cause of morbidity and mortality. Cardiovascular deaths are increased up to 4-fold in diabetics compared with their nondiabetic counterparts [1]. More than two-thirds of diabetics are obese. They require drugs that stimulate beta cells to make more insulin and/or drugs that help insulin work better. When these no longer work, people require insulin. Unfortunately, this form of diabetes is growing at an alarming rate. Since these patients will receive antidiabetic therapy indefinitely, any undesirable cardiovascular effects from well-known and widely used oral antidiabetic drugs should be analyzed in depth. In 1970, the University Group Diabetes Program (UGDP) reported a higher frequency of major cardiovascular events in patients with type 2 diabetes treated with tolbutamide, a sulfonylurea [2]. Awareness of this issue has increased during recent years following detection of the harmful influences of sulfonylureas on the ischemic myocardial cell [3, 4]. On the other hand, cardiovascular derangement associated with the use of metformin has also been reported during both short- [5, 6] and long-term follow-up [7].

When oral antidiabetic monotherapy does not achieve the glycemic goal, combination treatment is implemented. A sulfonylurea – usually glibenclamide (known also as glyburide in the USA) – plus metformin constitutes the most widely used antihyperglycemic combination in clinical practice [8]. However, the safety of this therapeutic regimen in long-term treatment is questionable [9]. The use of insulin in type 2 diabetes is also controversial. Nonetheless, after 15 or 20 years of disease, the majority of patients receive insulin [10]. The issue whether the adverse cardiovascular effects of each of these medications may be additive and detrimental for the coronary patient is of paramount importance but has not yet been addressed specifically.

Insulin resistance represents the background of a series of common factors for the development of both diabetes and heart disease. These factors include genetics, hypertension, obesity, hyperglycemia, dyslipidemia, prothrombotic state, aging, and physical inactivity. Once both diseases are clinically established, antidiabetic therapy per se may lead to a further derangement of cardiovascular status. Five types of oral antihperglycemic drugs are currently approved for the treatment of diabetes: biguanides, sulfonylureas, meglitinides, glitazones and alpha-glucosidase inhibitors. We will briefly review the cardiovascular effects of the most commonly used antidiabetic drugs within these types in an attempt to improve the knowledge and awareness regarding their influences and potential risks when treating patients with CAD, and review the current and potential research paths.

Biguanides

Metformin is the only drug belonging to the biguanide class currently available in most parts of the world. It reduces blood glucose levels through suppression of gluconeogenesis, stimulation of peripheral glucose uptake by tissue (mainly skeletal muscles) in the presence of insulin, and decreased absorption of glucose from the gastrointestinal tract. It has no direct effects on beta cells, does not produce hypoglycemia, reduces glycohemoglobin and improves both blood lipid profile and fibrinolytic activity. In contrast to other antidiabetic medications, metformin does not cause weight gain and appears to be the drug of choice in obese patients.

Despite these beneficial effects, metformin presents disadvantages that may influence the cardiovascular system. Gastrointestinal disturbances such as diarrhea are frequent, and the intestinal absorption of group B vitamins and folate is impaired during chronic therapy [15]. This deficiency may lead to increased plasma homocysteine levels which, in turn, accelerate the progression of vascular disease due to adverse effects on platelets, clotting factors, and endothelium [16] The existence of a graded association between homocysteine levels and overall mortality in patients with CAD is well established [16]. In addition, metformin may lead to lethal lactic acidosis, especially in patients with clinical conditions that predispose to this complication, such as heart failure or recent myocardial infarction [6]. It should be remembered that another drug of the biguanide group, phenformin, was withdrawn in many countries during the 1970s due to its link to lactic acidosis. A possible association of phenformin with increased cardiovascular mortality has also been suggested [17]. Finally, metformin undergoes renal excretion, presenting undesirable pharmacologic interactions with several widely used cardiovascular drugs. The coadministration of nifedipine or furosemide leads to increased metformin plasma levels. Furthermore, digoxin, quinidine, and triamterene – which are eliminated by renal tubular secretion – may interact with metformin by competing for proximal renal tubular transport systems [18]. Metformin was introduced in the USA in 1995, and serious controversies regarding cardiovascular safety followed its approval for use [5]. We have found increased mortality in CAD patients receiving metformin after a 5-year follow-up [7]. However, it should be stressed that this finding ought be treated with caution since it arose from a nonrandomized study in which information on drug doses and severity and duration of diabetes was incomplete or unavailable. In addition, metformin was found to be associated with less morbidity than sulfonylurea therapy in patients with diabetes and heart failure [19].

Sulfonylureas

These compounds have been available for nearly half a century. Today, sulfonylureas continue to represent a mainstay of therapy in patients with type 2 diabetes; their hypoglycemic potency is directly related to baseline plasma glucose values [20]. At the cellular level, they exert their action by closing the ATP-dependent potassium channels; this feature is responsible for both the insulinotropic effect and the adverse effects on the heart [3, 4]. Namely, sulfonylureas bind with high affinity to a subunit of these channels leading to depolarization of the cell. Under physiologic conditions, the channels remain closed. During ischemia, sulfonylureas may prevent their opening, avoiding the necessary hyperpolarization that protects the cell by impeding calcium influx [4]. In this context, it should be stressed that cardiac and vascular sulfonylurea receptors are structurally different from their pancreatic analog [4]. In fact, sulfonylureas have been reported to reduce resting myocardial blood flow [21], impair the recovery of contractile function after experimental ischemia [22], increase the ultimate infarct size [23], elicit proarrhythmic effects [24], abolish ischemic preconditioning in animal models [25], and increase early mortality in patients with diabetes mellitus after direct angioplasty for acute myocardial infarction [26]. Prevention of myocardial preconditioning by glibenclamide has also been demonstrated in clinical trials [27].

It is important to stress that not all the undesirable effects on cardiovascular outcome reported for the first-generation sulfonylureas such as tolbutamide [2] can be automatically extrapolated to the more modern second-generation compounds such as glibenclamide, which is short-acting and possesses antiarrhythmic properties [3]. In our experience, cardiovascular mortality rates in CAD patients on sulfonylureas (mainly glibenclamide) were lower than those on combined sulfonylurea-metformin therapy, and similar to the rates in patients on diet alone [7]. Another new second-generation sulfonylurea, glimepiride, is more pancreas-specific and does not show interaction with cardiovascular ATP-dependent potassium channels [3, 27].

Meglitinides

Meglitinides stimulate insulin secretion. The first drug of this group, repaglinide, a benzoic acid derivative, was introduced in the USA in 1998. The second, nateglinide, is a *d*-phenylalanine derivative. Like sulfonylureas, these compounds act by closing the ATP-dependent potassium channels. However, its mechanism of action seem to be more complex since possibly three meglitinide receptor-binding sites have been found on the beta cells [28].

Despite a common basic mechanism of action, the insulinotropic effects of the two approved agents can be influenced differently by ambient glucose, leading to dissimilar responsiveness. Nateglinide may exert a more physiologic effect on insulin secretion, i.e. a glycemia-dependent response, than repaglinide, presenting less propensity to elicit hypoglycemia in vivo [29]. On the other hand, nateglinide presents a relatively lesser influence on glycohemoglobin levels. When used as monotherapy, these drugs reduce both fasting plasma glucose and glycohemoglobin, and have no significant effects on the lipid profile. They present some specific characteristics that differentiate them from sulfonylureas: pills are taken before meals (the medication should not be administered if a meal is skipped), exhibit a short onset of action and a short pharmacologic half-life, and act mainly on postprandial glucose.

The cardiovascular safety of these insulin secretagogues is still uncertain. Increased morbidity, particularly acute ischemic events, was observed for repaglinide after 1 year compared with glibenclamide. Nevertheless, patients on repaglinide appeared to have had more severe CAD at baseline than those in the glibenclamide group, and when adjustments were made the relative risk declined [30]. Thus, while definite assertions regarding cardiovascular safety cannot be made at this stage, caution should be implemented in view of the strong involvement of the ATP-dependent potassium channels in the mechanism of action.

Glitazones

This group of drugs was introduced in 1997 and includes antidiabetic medications such as troglitazone, pioglitazone, and rosiglitazone, the chemical structure and mechanisms of action of which are very different from those of the other groups. Chemically, they are thiazolidinediones having chroman moieties; some of the analogues may present an aminoalkyl group as a linker between the chroman ring and the 4-[5-(2,4-dioxo-1, 3-thiazolidinyl)methyl] phenoxy moiety. Troglitazone, which was the first agent in this class to receive labeling approval, was withdrawn from clinical use in the US due to hepatotoxicity [31].

These recently developed drugs are insulin sensitizers, and they bind to a novel receptor called peroxisome proliferator-activated receptor (PPAR)-gamma, leading to increased glucose transporter expression. Sensitivity to insulin – especially in adipocytes, muscle and liver – is improved, and an additional major effect is the inhibition of hepatic gluconeogenesis [32]. It should be pointed out that no increment in insulin secretion is documented. PPARs are transcription factors belonging to the superfamily of nuclear receptors; nowadays, three isoforms (alpha, beta/delta, gamma) are known, which regulate glucose homeostasis, lipoprotein metabolism, local immune responses, local inflammation, tumor development and thrombosis and also present potential antiatherogenic effects [33].

Glitazone monotherapy is only modestly effective in reducing glucose and glycohemoglobin levels. Plasma triglycerides are reduced by 10–20%, and HDL cholesterol levels increase by 5–10%, since glitazones also stimulates the isoform PPAR-alpha that regulates lipid metabolism. These favorable effects are counterbalanced by a 10–15% increase in LDL cholesterol [11]. Edema has been reported in 5% of patients, and these drugs are contraindicated in diabetics with NYHA class III or IV cardiac status [11]. Regarding hepatotoxicity, studies with rosiglitazone and pioglitazone indicate that it is not a class effect. Further differences in the safety profiles of these agents arise because the oxidative metabolism for each agent occurs by distinct cytochrome pathways: pioglitazone involves CYP 3A4 and CYP 2C8 whereas rosiglitazone is principally metabolized by CYP 2C8. CYP 3A4 is involved in the metabolism of over 150 drugs, hence the potential for drug interactions with pioglitazone is much greater than with rosiglitazone. Class effects include slight reductions in hemoglobin and hematocrit (due to hemodilution) [31].

It was stressed that rosiglitazone reduces urinary albumin excretion in type 2 diabetes and may even mildly reduce blood pressure [34]. Nontraditional markers of cardiovascular disease – such as matrix metalloproteinase-9 – may also be reduced [35]. In addition, another notorious characteristic of glitazones is their capability of lowering leptin levels, leading to several degrees of weight gain, usually proportional to the administered dose [34]. This feature has obvious harmful clinical implications and was documented in both experimental [36, 37] and human studies [35]. In addition, it was recently suggested that rosiglitazone may be associated with a significant increase in the risk of myocardial infarction and with an increase in the risk of death from cardiovascular causes that had borderline significance [38].

Thus, glitazones exhibit a broad landscape of complex clinical effects, in part favorable and in part detrimental for the cardiovascular system. The concluding balance between these effects requires further elucidation.

Alpha-Glucosidase Inhibitors

The primary mechanism of action of some novel antidiabetic drugs like acarbose, voglibose and miglitol is grounded on competitive inhibition of several enzymes of the alpha-glucosidase group (maltase, isomaltase, sucrase, glucoamylase). These are membrane-bound enzymes that hydrolyze oligosaccharides and disaccharides to glucose in the brush border of the small intestine Thus, by delaying the digestion of carbohydrates, these compounds shift their absorption to more distal parts of the small intestine and colon, and defer gastrointestinal absorption of glucose. Their hypoglycemic potency is less than that of biguanides and sulfonylureas [11] and, unlike the latter, they do not cause hypoglycemia. The most frequent side effects of these drugs are mild abdominal pain, flatulence and diarrhea [39].

It is well established that impaired fasting glucose concentrations in nondiabetic patients with ischemic heart disease are a marker for a worse prognosis [40, 41]. Acarbose could be used, either as an alternative or in addition to changes in lifestyle, to delay the development of type 2 diabetes in these patients [39]. The long-term effects of these agents on morbidity and mortality rates and on diabetic micro- and macrovascular complications have not yet been studied [42].

Combined Antihyperglycemic Treatment

Combined therapy is based on the premise that pharmacological agents acting via different mechanisms and presenting differing side effects permit the design of individualized antidiabetic regimens. This approach reflects the plausibility that monotherapy with any currently available medication is likely to fail over time in some patients, and this type of pharmacological diabetes management is widely used. Recent findings from the UKPDS showed that after 3 years, approximately 50% of patients could attain satisfactory glucose levels with monotherapy; by 9 years this had declined to only 25% [43]. Long-term problem-oriented prospective studies that focus specifically on the outcome of coronary diabetics on combined therapy are lacking. Data from an observational study – which included exclusively documented coronary patients – performed at our laboratory [44] indicate an all-cause increased crude mortality over a mean 7.7-year follow-up in diabetics on combined treatment with metformin and glibenclamide. These results were corroborated when multivariate analysis was performed. Another study that focused on the general diabetic population found that there was an higher cardiovascular mortality in type 2 diabetics taking sulfonylurea and metformin in combination than in those taking only sulfonylurea [45], concluding that it cannot be excluded that this kind of combination therapy possibly increases cardiovascular mortality. Combination therapy is known to promote additional blood glucose reduction but there is as yet no evidence that these or another antidiabetic formulations are beneficial in preventing or delaying macrovascular disease. These observations are in keeping with the United Kingdom Prospective Diabetes Study (UKPDS) reports demonstrating excess risk of all-cause mortality in the whole diabetic population receiving combined therapy, especially in patients in whom metformin was added at an early stage [46].

Hence, the combined antihyperglycemic treatment leads to a peculiar entanglement since sulfonylureas and metformin are (1) the most powerful antiabetic drugs; (2) those presenting the most unfavorable cardiac effects, and (3) the most frequently employed combination in routine clinical practice.

Clinical Implications

As we enter the 21st century, our pharmacological armamentarium is increasingly complex, offering a wide array of drugs, both as monotherapy or in combination. It is therefore frequently difficult to determine the best therapeutic option for a given patient. A common problem arises when a drug is known to give a prompt and beneficial effect in the short term, but data regarding long-term outcome and safety are either lacking or insufficient. This is particularly true regarding antihyperglycemic drugs in patients with CAD.

Comprehensive risk reduction is mandatory for diabetic patients with CAD. General measures should comprise diet, physical activity, complete cessation of smoking, and weight and lipid profile management. However, fewer than 10% of patients achieve acceptable long-term glycemic values with non-pharmacological therapy only [47]. Special emphasis should be given to blood pressure control; we have reported the presence of widespread undiagnosed hypertension in this population, which presented a 5-year mortality even higher than that in diabetics previously identified as hypertensives [48]. Moreover, the increased mortality associated with hypertension in mild diet-treated type 2 diabetes strongly supports the need for early onset of antihypertensive treatment in these patients [49]. When examining the status of glucose metabolism in patients with heart failure secondary to coronary artery disease, it is disclosed that both type 2 diabetes and impaired fasting glucose are associated with increased prevalence of heart failure among patients with CAD [50].

Evidence is available that long-term maintenance of normal or near-normal glucose levels using pharmacological means is protective in diabetics, improving microvascular disease (retinopathy, nephropathy, and neuropathy) and reducing both morbidity and mortality [51]. Taking into consideration that several degrees of undesirable cardiovascular effects have been reported for most antidiabetic drugs, is this also applicable to coronary diabetics? Current data indicate that the answer is yes, but alleviation of macrovascular complications remains dubious and the therapeutic criteria should not be automatically extrapolated to CAD patients, who need carefully customized treatment.

We believe that an oral antihyperglycemic agent, for example a sulfonylurea, or metformin in obese patients, should constitute first-line pharmacological therapy in type 2 diabetics with CAD; this is in keeping with the recommendations of the American Heart Association [52]. As second-line therapy, ancillary medications such as alpha-glucosidase inhibitors could be added if target glucose levels are not achieved, but glibenclamide and metformin should not be used together. Finally, there is no contraindication to add insulin at a later stage as third-line therapy, provided the risk of hyperinsulinemic hypoalphalipoproteinemia – especially when associated with low HDL cholesterol levels – is monitored [53].

What should the policy be regarding the widely used sulfonylurea-metformin combined treatment? Following approval of a given therapy for a chronic condition, large prospective, randomized, placebo-controlled trials designed to check its long-term safety and effectiveness require many years to be completed, and sometimes such studies are not performed at all. This is the case with this combined treatment in CAD patients. The data available at present indicate increased mortality in patients receiving this therapy [44–46, 54], suggesting that this combination should be used with caution in diabetics with proven CAD. The excessive mortality rate could reflect an additive expression of the adverse cardiovascular effects of each of these medications. However, we would like to stress that our own observations specifically address glibenclamide-metformin combined treatment [42] and we have no information regarding combinations of metformin with other sulfonylureas such as glimepiride or gliclazide. Thus, we consider that:

(1) Four of the five oral antidiabetic drug groups present proven or potential cardiac hazards.
(2) These hazards are not mere 'side effects', but phenomena which are deeply rooted in the drugs' mechanism of action.
(3) Current data indicate that combined glibenclamide/metformin therapy seems to present a special risk and should be avoided in the long-term management of type 2 diabetics with proven CAD.
(4) Customized antihyperglycemic pharmacological approaches should be investigated for the achievement of optimal treatment of diabetic patients with heart disease [54].

Current and Future Research Paths

Taking into consideration the intimate interrelationship between diabetes and heart disease, in 1999 the American Heart Association coined the phrase 'diabetes is a cardiovascular disease' [52]. Diabetic patients with CAD connote an enormous population which deserves a specific approach. Incretins and dipeptidyl peptidase (DPP)-4 inhibitors represent novel pharmacological approaches.

Incretins

Incretin mimetic drugs are nowadays extensively investigated. A key role for intestinal peptides in the regulation of postprandial insulin secretion and glucose levels was proposed, based on the observation that insulin responses to an oral glucose load exceeded those measured after intravenous administration of an equivalent amount of glucose [55]. This phenomenon, termed the 'incretin effect', postulated the existence of gut-derived signals promoting insulin secretion in response to nutrient intake [56]. Subsequently, the incretin hormones, gastric inhibitory polypeptide (GIP, renamed glucose-dependent insulinotropic peptide) and glucagon-like peptide-1 (GLP-1), were discovered [57]. These two principal incretin hormones are small peptides, 42 and 30 amino acids, respectively, that rapidly stimulate the release of insulin only when blood glucose levels are elevated, thereby enhancing the glucose-sensing and insulin secretory capacity of the endocrine pancreas during postprandial hyperglycemia [58].

The physiological actions of incretins have been extensively defined in animal studies with exogenous GLP-1 and GLP-1 receptor antagonists, highlighting its role as a meal-stimulated factor with potent glucose-lowering activity. Of significant clinical relevance is that exogenous GLP-1 has the potential to normalize fasting plasma glucose concentrations in patients with type 2 diabetes. In several studies in subjects with diabetes, GLP-1 – whether administered by intravenous or subcutaneous infusion – normalized both fasting and postprandial glycemia by enhancing glucose-mediated insulin secretion, as well as by suppressing glucagon secretion [59–62].

Additional studies in animals and humans have demonstrated glucose-lowering effects of GLP-1. GLP-1 slows gastric emptying to decrease the rate of nutrient absorption, which results in more synchronous nutrient delivery with endogenous insulin action. Significant acute reductions in appetite and food intake after intravenous administration of GLP-1 in both healthy individuals and in patients with type 2 diabetes have also been demonstrated [63–65].

The mechanism through which the incretin hormones elicit their cytoprotective effects on the beta cell has attracted significant attention because preservation and restoration of beta cell mass may contribute to the therapeutic potential of the incretins for the treatment of both type 1 and type 2 diabetes. Endoplasmic reticulum stress within the beta cell, possibly occurring as a result of the overproduction or misfolding of insulin, may be a contributing factor to increased beta cell apoptosis and the loss of islet mass observed in diabetic patients [66].

Exenatide was first in the new class of incretin mimetics for the treatment of patients with type 2 diabetes. Several short-term phase 2 clinical trials in patients with type 2 diabetes have reported that subcutaneous exenatide acutely lowered both fasting and postprandial plasma glucose concentrations. The rate of gastric emptying was also slowed in patients treated with exenatide. Large-scale clinical trials designed to assess the safety and efficacy of twice-daily sub-cutaneous exenatide over a 6-month period were completed in subjects with type 2 diabetes who were unable to attain glycemic control with oral sulfony-lureas, metformin, or both [67].

Another incretin mimetic compound, liraglutide, is a once-daily GLP-1 derivative which is in development for the treatment of type 2 diabetes. GLP-1, in its natural form, is short-lived in the body (the half-life after subcutaneous injection is approximately 1 h), so it is not very useful as a therapeutic agent. However, liraglutide is a 'timed release' form of GLP-1 with prolonged activity; the half-life after subcutaneous injection is 11–15 h, making it suitable for once-daily dosing. This prolonged action is achieved by attaching a fatty acid molecule at one position of the GLP-1 molecule, enabling it to bind to albumin within the subcutaneous tissue and bloodstream. The active GLP-1 is then released from albumin at a slow, consistent rate. Binding with albumin also results in slower degradation and reduced elimination of liraglutide from the circulation by the kidneys compared to GLP-1 in its natural form [68, 69].

Dipeptidyl Peptidase (DPP)-4 Inhibitors

DPP-4 is a ubiquitously expressed serine protease that exhibits postproline or alanine peptidase activity, thereby generating biologically inactive peptides via cleavage at the N-terminal region after X-proline or X-alanine. It is a com-plex molecule that exists as a membrane-spanning cell-anchored protein that is expressed on many cell types, and as a soluble form in the circulation; both forms have proteolytic activity. Because both GLP-1 and GIP have an alanine residue at position 2, they are substrates for DPP-4. DPP-4 inhibitors like sitagliptin are orally administered drugs that improve glycemic control by pre-venting the rapid degradation of incretin hormones, thereby resulting in post-prandial increases in levels of biologically active intact GLP-1 and GIP [70, 71].

Sitagliptin is an orally bioavailable selective DPP-4 inhibitor that was dis-covered through the optimization of a class of beta amino acid-derived DPP-4 inhibitors. It lowers DPP-4 activity in a sustained manner following once daily administration, preserves the circulating levels of intact GIP and GLP1 following meals in both acute and chronic studies and reduces blood glucose levels without significant increases in hypoglycemia [72]. Thus, the drug works by inhibiting the inactivation of the incretin GLP-1 and GIP by DPP-4. By preventing GLP-1 and GIP inactivation, GLP-1 and GIP are able to potentiate the secretion of insulin and suppress the release of glucagon by the pancreas.

Several additional DPP-4 inhibitors, like saxagliptin and vildagliptin, are currently investigated. Their beneficial effects are that they (1) increase circulating levels of GLP-1 in animals and humans, (2) increase the genesis, proliferation and differentiation of beta cells, (3) inhibit apoptosis of these cells, (4) enhance insulin secretion, (5) reduce fasting glucose, (6) reduce postparandial glucoser, and (7) reduce HbA1c levels.

In comparison to DPP-4 inhibitors, incretin mimetic agents have more pharmacological specificity but require subcutaneous injections. As with DPP-4 inhibitors, improvements in glycemic control were achieved with either no weight gain or with weight loss. Considering the impact of obesity on diabetes, along with weight gain that generally accompanies the use of insulin, insulin secretagogues, and insulin sensitizers, interventions with positive effects on weight are likely to become increasingly important.

Cardiovascular adverse effects were not described for these compounds, targeting them as an ideal combined therapy for diabetic patients with heart disease.

Additional Therapeutic Paths

Future paths of antidiabetic pharmacological investigation should focus on both longitudinal problem-oriented long-term epidemiological studies and on research in molecular biology. An important area of research would be to further scrutinize the structural and functional differences between pancreatic and cardiac isoforms of ATP-dependent potassium channels. This would allow development of specific insulinotropic compounds that interact exclusively with the pancreatic channel, leaving the cardiac channel unaffected [4, 27].

The development of newer insulin compounds represents an additional path of intensive current research. Since the discovery of insulin, subcutaneous injection has been the only possible mode of administration due to the massive degradation of orally administered insulin by proteases in the gastrointestinal tract. The subcutaneous route leads to unphysiologically high insulin levels in peripheral blood relative to those achieved in the portal vein, besides being cumbersome and painful. A recent development aimed at partially overcoming these problems is insulin glargine, a long-acting analogue created by the recombinant DNA modification of human insulin. Injected once daily, it provides a relatively constant basal level of circulating insulin with no pronounced peak, is well tolerated and elicits less hypoglycemia, especially nocturnal episodes, than NPH insulin, with similar levels of glycemic control [73].

An additional interesting progress is inhaled insulin. The lung presents inherent advantages for insulin administration, which include a vast and well-perfused absorptive surface, absence of some peptidases that are present in the digestive tract, and a thin alveolar-capillary barrier [74]. The optimal particle size for pulmonary insulin appears to be in the range of 2–5 μm; these sizes allow deposition in the alveoli. Larger particles will precipitate on the oropharynx or bronchial mucous membranes, while smaller ones will be exhaled. The inhalation of insulin particles results in a time-action profile characterized by a faster onset than regular subcutaneous insulin [75]. Compared with patients who only received insulin injections, patients receiving inhaled insulin experienced significant reductions in both fasting plasma glucose levels and 2-hour postprandial glucose levels. Concerns have been raised about the safety of the preparation and whether it will compromise lung capacity or damage lung tissue in long-term use. However, in clinical trials the frequency and nature of adverse events were similar in the active and the control groups [76].

Finally, oral insulin compounds have been investigated and constitute a promising field. Significant improvements of oral insulin absorption were already attained by masking the hydrophilic surface of its molecule. Moreover, chemical modification of the molecule by optimizing the fatty acid chain length with palmitic acid achieved an enhanced oral absorption of insulin [77–79].

References

1   Wigard DL, Barrett-Connor E: Heart disease and diabetes; in Harris MI, Cowie CC, Stern MP, Boyko EJ, Reiber GE, Bennett PH (eds): Diabetes in America, ed 2. Washington, US Government Printing Office, 1995, pp 429–448.
2   Klimt CR, Knatterud GL, Meinert CL, Prout TE: The University Group Diabetes Program: a study of the effect of hypoglycemic agents on vascular complications in patients with adult-onset diabetes. I. Design, methods and baseline characteristics. II. Mortality results. Diabetes 1970;19 (suppl 2):747–830.
3   Smits P, Thien T: Cardiovascular effects of sulphonylurea derivatives: implication for the treatment of NIDDM? Diabetologia 1995;38:116–121.
4   Brady PA, Terzic A: The sulfonylurea controversy: more questions from the heart. J Am Coll Cardiol 1998;31:950–956.
5   Innerfield RJ: Metformin-associated mortality in US studies. N Engl J Med 1996;334:1611–1613.
6   Misbin RI, Green L, Stadel BV, Gueriguian JL, Gubbi A, Fleming GA: Lactic acidosis in patients with diabetes treated with metformin. N Engl J Med 1998;338:265–266.
7   Fisman EZ, Tenenbaum A, Benderly M, Goldbourt U, Behar S, Motro M: Antihyperglycemic treatment in diabetics with coronary disease: increased metformin-associated mortality over a 5-year follow-up. Cardiology 1999;91:195–202.
8   Consensus Statement: The pharmacological treatment of hyperglycemia in NIDDM. Diabetes Care 1996;19(suppl I):S54–S61.
9   Nathan DM: Some answers, more controversy, from UKPDS. Lancet 1998;352:832–833.

10 Fertig BJ, Simmons DA, Martin DB: Therapy for diabetes; in Harris MI, Cowie CC, Stern MP, Boyko EJ, Reiber GE, Bennett PH (eds): Diabetes in America, ed 2. Washington, US Government Printing Office, 1995, pp 519–539.

11 DeFronzo RA: Pharmacologic therapy for type 2 diabetes. Ann Intern Med 1999;131:281–303.

12 Taylor SI, Accili D, Imai Y: Perspectives in diabetes: insulin resistance or insulin deficiency: which is the primary cause of NIDDM? Diabetes 1994;43:735–740.

13 University Group Diabetes Program: Effects of hypoglycemic agents on vascular complications in patients with adult-onset diabetes. VII. Evaluation of insulin therapy: final report. Diabetes 1982;31(suppl 5):1–78.

14 Adler AI, Neil HAW, Manley SE, Holman RR, Turner CT: Hyperglycemia and hyperinsulinemia at diagnosis of diabetes and their association with subsequent cardiovascular disease in the United Kingdom Prospective Diabetes Study (UKPDS 47). Am Heart J 1999;138:S353–S359.

15 Adams JF, Clark JS, Ireland JT, Kesson CM, Watson WS: Malabsorption of vitamin B_{12} and intrinsic factor secretion during biguanide therapy. Diabetologia 1983;24:16–18.

16 Mayer EL, Jacobsen DW, Robinson K: Homocysteine and coronary atherosclerosis. J Am Coll Cardiol 1996;27:517–527.

17 Goldner MG, Knatterud GL, Prout TE: Effects of hypoglycemic agents on vascular complications in patients with adult-onset diabetes. III. Clinical implication of UGDP results. JAMA 1971;218:1400–1410.

18 Marchetti P, Navalesi R: Pharmacokinetic-pharmacodynamic relationships of oral hypoglycemic agents: an update. Clin Pharmacokinet 1989;16:100–128.

19 Eurich DT, Majumdar SR, McAlister FA, Tsuyuki RT, Johnson JA: Improved clinical outcomes associated with metformin in patients with diabetes and heart failure. Diabetes Care 2005;28:2345–2351.

20 Rosenstock J, Samols E, Muchmore DB, Schneider J: Glimepiride, a new once-daily sulfonylurea: a double-blind placebo-controlled study of NIDDM patients. Glimepiride Study Group. Diabetes Care 1996;19:1194–1199.

21 Duncker DJ, van Zon NS, Altman JD, Pavek DJ, Bache RJ: Role of K+ ATP channels in coronary vasodilation during exercise. Circulation 1993;88:1245–1253.

22 Cole WC, McPherson CD, Sontag D: ATP-regulated K^+ channels protect the myocardium against ischemia/reperfusion damage. Circ Res 1991;69:571–581.

23 Toombs CF, McGee DS, Johnston WE, Vinten-Johansen J: Myocardial protective effects of adenosine: infarct size reduction with pretreatment and continued receptor stimulation during ischemia. Circulation 1992;86:986–994.

24 Pogatsa G, Koltai ZM, Ballagi-Pordany G: Influence of hypoglycemic sulfonylurea compounds on the incidence of ventricular ectopic beats in non-insulin-dependent diabetic patients treated with digitalis. Curr Ther Res 1993;53:329–339.

25 Grover GJ, Sleph PG, Dzwonick BS: Role of myocardial ATP-sensitive potassium channels in mediating preconditioning in the dog heart and their possible interactions with adenosine A1-receptors. Circulation 1992;86:1310–1316.

26 Garratt KN, Brady PA, Hassinger NL, Grill DE, Terzic A, Holmes DR: Sulfonylurea drugs increase early mortality in patients with diabetes mellitus after direct angioplasty for acute myocardial infarction. J Am Coll Cardiol 1999;33:119–124.

27 Klepzig H, Kober G, Matter C, Luus H, Schneider H, Boedeker KH, Kiowski W, Amann FW, Gruber D, Harris S, Burger W: Sulfonylureas and ischemic preconditioning: a double-blind, placebo-controlled evaluation of glimepiride and glibenclamide. Eur Heart J 1999;20:439–446.

28 Fuhlendorff J, Rorsman P, Kofod H, Brand CL, Rolin B, MacKay P: Stimulation of insulin release by repaglinide and glibenclamide involves both common and distinct processes. Diabetes 1998;47:345–351.

29 Hu S, Wang S, Dunning BE: Glucose-dependent and glucose-sensitizing insulinotropic effect of nateglinide: comparison to sulfonylureas and repaglinide. Int J Exp Diabetes Res 2001;2:63–72.

30 Fleming A: FDA approach to the regulation of drugs for diabetes. Am Heart J 1999;138: S339–S345.

31 Lebovitz HE: Differentiating members of the thiazolidinedione class: a focus on safety. Diabetes Metab Res Rev 2002;18(suppl 2):S23–S29.

32   Saltiel AR, Olefsky JM: Thiazolidinediones in the treatment of insulin resistance and type II diabetes. Diabetes 1996;45:1661–1669.

33   Duval C, Chinetti G, Trottein F, Fruchart JC, Staels B: The role of PPARs in atherosclerosis. Trends Mol Med 2002;8:422–430.

34   Bakris G, Viberti G, Weston WM, Heise M, Porter LE, Freed MI: Rosiglitazone reduces urinary albumin excretion in type 2 diabetes. J Hum Hypertens 2003;17:7–12.

35   Haffner SM, Greenberg AS, Weston WM, Chen H, Williams K, Freed MI: Effect of rosiglitazone treatment on nontraditional markers of cardiovascular disease in patients with type 2 diabetes mellitus. Circulation 2002;106:679–684.

36   Goetze S, Bungenstock A, Czupalla C, Eilers F, Stawowy P, Kintscher U, Spencer-Hansch C, Graf K, Nurnberg B, Law RE, Fleck E, Grafe M: Leptin induces endothelial cell migration through Akt, which is inhibited by PPAR gamma-ligands. Hypertension 2002;40:748–754.

37   Nisoli E, Carruba MO, Tonello C, Macor C, Federspil G, Vettor R: Induction of fatty acid translocase/CD36, peroxisome proliferator-activated receptor-gamma2, leptin, uncoupling proteins 2 and 3, and tumor necrosis factor-alpha gene expression in human subcutaneous fat by lipid infusion. Diabetes 2000;49:319–324.

38   Nissen SE, Wolski K: Effect of rosiglitazone on the risk of myocardial infarction and death from cardiovascular causes. N Engl J Med 2007;356:2457–2471.

39   Chiasson JL, Josse RG, Gomis R, Hanefeld M, Karasik A, Laakso M, STOP-NIDDM Trail Research Group: Acarbose for prevention of type 2 diabetes mellitus: the STOP-NIDDM randomised trial. Lancet 2002;359:2072–2077.

40   Fisman EZ, Motro M, Tenenbaum A, Boyko V, Mandelzweig L, Behar S: Impaired fasting glucose concentrations in nondiabetic patients with ischemic heart disease: a marker for a worse prognosis. Am Heart J 2001;141:485–490.

41   Tenenbaum A, Motro M, Fisman EZ, Boyko V, Mandelzweig L, Reicher-Reiss H, Graff E, Brunner D, Behar S: Clinical impact of borderline and undiagnosed diabetes mellitus in patients with coronary artery disease. Am J Cardiol 2000;86:1363–1366.

42   Rao SV, Bethel MA, Feinglos MN: Treatment of diabetes mellitus: implications of the use of oral agents. Am Heart J 1999;138:S334–S337.

43   Turner RC, Cull CA, Frighi V, Holman RR: Glycemic control with diet, sulfonylurea, metformin or insulin in patients with type 2 diabetes: progressive requirement for multiple therapies (UKPDS 49). UK Diabetes Prospective Study (UKPDS) Group. JAMA 1999;281:2005–2012.

44   Fisman EZ, Tenenbaum A, Boyko V, Benderly M, Adler Y, Friedensohn A, Kohanovski M, Rotzak R, Schneider H, Behar S, Motro M: Oral antidiabetic treatment in patients with coronary disease: time-related increased mortality on combined glyburide/metformin therapy over a 7.7-year follow-up. Clin Cardiol 2001;24:151–158.

45   Olsson J, Lindberg G, Gottsater M, Lindwall K, Sjostrand A, Tisell A, Melander A: Increased mortality in type II diabetic patients using sulphonylurea and metformin in combination: a population-based observational study. Diabetologia 2000;43:558–560.

46   UK Diabetes Prospective Study (UKPDS) Group: Effect of intensive blood-gucose control on complications in overweight patients with type 2 diabetes (UKPDS 34). Lancet 1998;352: 854–865.

47   Giugliano D: Does treatment of noninsulin-dependent diabetes mellitus reduce the risk of coronary heart disease? Curr Opinion Lipidol 1996;7:227–233.

48   Tenenbaum A, Fisman EZ, Boyko V, Goldbourt U, Auerbach I, Shemesh J, Shotan A, Reicher-Reiss H, Behar S, Motro M: Prevalence and prognostic significance of unrecognized systemic hypertension in patients with diabetes mellitus and healed myocardial infarction and/or stable angina pectoris. Am J Cardiol 1999;84:294–298.

49   Tenenbaum A, Fisman EZ, Boyko V, Goldbourt U, Graff E, Shemesh J, Shotan A, Reicher-Reiss H, Behar S, Motro M: Hypertension in diet versus pharmacologically treated diabetics: mortality over a 5-year follow-up. Hypertension 1999;33:1002–1007.

50   Tenenbaum A, Motro M, Fisman EZ, Leor J, Boyko V, Mandelzweig L, Behar S: Status of glucose metabolism in patients with heart failure secondary to coronary artery disease. Am J Cardiol 2002;90:529–532.

51 The American Association of Clinical Endocrinologists Medical Guidelines for the Management of Diabetes Mellitus: The AACE System of intensive diabetes self-management – 1999 update. Endocr Pract 2000;6:1–44.

52 Grundy SM, Benjamin IJ, Burke GL, Chait A, Eckel RH, Howard BV, Mitch W, Smith SC, Sowers JR: Diabetes and cardiovascular disease: a statement for healthcare professionals from the American Heart Association. Circulation 1999;100:1134–1146.

53 Saku K, Zhang B, Shirai K, Jimi S, Yoshinaga K, Arakawa K: Hyperinsulinemic hypoalphalipoproteinemia as a new indicator for coronary artery disease. J Am Coll Cardiol 1999;31: 1443–1451.

54 Fisman EZ, Tenenbaum A, Motro M, Adler Y: Oral antidiabetic therapy in patients with heart disease: a cardiologic standpoint. Herz 2004;29:290–298.

55 Perley M, Kipnis DM: Plasma insulin responses to oral and intravenous glucose: studies in normal and diabetic subjects. J Clin Invest 1967;46:1954–1962.

56 Nauck MA, Homberger E, Siegel EG, Allen RC, Eaton RP, Ebert R, Creutzfeldt W: Incretin effects of increasing glucose loads in man calculated from venous insulin and C-peptide responses. J Clin Endocrinol Metab 1986;63:492–498.

57 Kreymann B, Williams G, Ghatei MA, Bloom SR: Glucagon-like peptide-1 736: a physiological incretin in man. Lancet 1987;ii:1300–1304.

58 Efendic S, Portwood N: Overview of incretin hormones. Horm Metab Res 2004;36:742–746.

59 Creutzfeldt WO, Kleine N, Willms B, Orskov C, Holst JJ, Nauck MA: Glucagonostatic actions and reduction of fasting hyperglycemia by exogenous glucagon-like peptide I(736) amide in type I diabetic patients. Diabetes Care 1996;19:580–586.

60 Nauck MA, Wollschlager D, Werner J, Holst JJ, Orskov C, Creutzfeldt W, Willms B: Effects of subcutaneous glucagon-like peptide 1 (GLP-1 [7–36 amide]) in patients with NIDDM. Diabetologia 1996;39:1546–1553.

61 Rachman J, Barrow BA, Levy JC, Turner RC: Near-normalisation of diurnal glucose concentrations by continuous administration of glucagon-like peptide-1 (GLP-1) in subjects with NIDDM. Diabetologia 1997;40:205–211.

62 Zander M, Madsbad S, Madsen JL, Holst JJ: Effect of 6-week course of glucagon-like peptide 1 on glycaemic control, insulin sensitivity, and beta-cell function in type 2 diabetes: a parallel-group study. Lancet 2002;359:824–830.

63 Vilsboll T, Holst JJ: Incretins, insulin secretion and type 2 diabetes mellitus. Diabetologia 2004;47: 357–366.

64 Nauck MA, Baller B, Meier JJ: Gastric inhibitory polypeptide and glucagon-like peptide-1 in the pathogenesis of type 2 diabetes. Diabetes 2004;53(suppl 3):S190–S196.

65 Deacon CF: Circulation and degradation of GIP and GLP-1. Horm Metab Res 2004;36:761–765.

66 Burcelin R: The incretins: a link between nutrients and well-being. Br J Nutr 2005;93(suppl 1): S147–S156.

67 Kendall DM, Riddle MC, Zhuang D, et al: Effects of exenatide (exendin-4) on glycemic control and weight in patients with type 2 diabetes treated with metformin and a sulfonylurea. Diabetologia 2004;47(suppl 1):A279–A280.

68 Rolin B, Larsen MO, Gotfredsen CF: The long-acting GLP-1 derivative NN2211 ameliorates glycemia and increases β-cell mass in diabetic mice. Am J Physiol 2002;283:E745–E752.

69 Agerso H, Jensen LB, Elbrond B, Rolan P, Zdravkovic M: The pharmacokinetics, pharmacodynamics, safety and tolerability of NN2211, a new long-acting GLP-1 derivative, in healthy men. Diabetologia 2002;45:195–202.

70 Drucker DJ: The biology of incretin hormones. Cell Metab 2006;3:153–165.

71 Drucker DJ: Therapeutic potential of dipeptidyl peptidase IV inhibitors for the treatment of type 2 diabetes. Expert Opin Invest Drugs 2003;12:87–100.

72 Kim D, Wang L, Beconi M, Eiermann GJ, Fisher MH, He H, Hickey GJ, Kowalchick JE, Leiting B, Lyons K, Marsilio F, McCann ME, Patel RA, Petrov A, Scapin G, Patel SB, Roy RS, Wu JK, Wyvratt MJ, Zhang BB, Zhu L, Thornberry NA, Weber AE: (2R)-4-oxo-4-[3-(trifluoromethyl)-5,6-dihydro[1,2,4]triazolo[4,3-a]pyrazin-7(8H)-yl]-1-(2,4,5-trifluorophenyl)butan-2-amine: a potent, orally active dipeptidyl peptidase IV inhibitor for the treatment of type 2 diabetes. J Med Chem 2005;48:141–151.

73 Owens DR, Griffiths S: Insulin glargine (Lantus). Int J Clin Pract 2002;56:460–466.
74 Heinemann L, Pfutzner A, Heise T: Alternative routes of administration as an approach to improve insulin therapy: update on dermal, oral, nasal and pulmonary insulin delivery. Curr Pharm Design 2001;7:1327–1351.
75 Heinemann L, Klappoth W, Rave K, Hompesch B, Linkeschowa R, Heise T: Intra-individual variability of the metabolic effect of inhaled insulin together with an absorption enhancer. Diabetes Care 2000;23:1343–1347.
76 Hegewald M, Crapo RO, Jensen RL: Pulmonary function changes related to acute and chronic administration of inhaled insulin. Diabetes Technol Ther 2007;9(suppl 1):S93–S101.
77 Hashizume M, Douen T, Murakami M, Yamamoto A, Takado K, Muranishi S: Improvement of large intestinal absorption of insulin by chemical modification with palmitic acid in rats. J Pharm Pharmcol 1992;44:555–559.
78 Mesiha MS, Plakogiannis F, Vejosoth S: Enhanced oral absorption of insulin from desolvated fatty acid-sodium glycocholate emulsion. Int J Pharm 1994;111:213–216.
79 Mesiha MS, Ponnapula P, Plakogiannis F: Oral absorption of insulin encapsulated in artificial chyles of bile salts, palmitic acid and alfa-tocopherol dispersions. Int J Pharm 2002;249:1–5.

Prof. Enrique Z. Fisman
Cardiovascular Diabetology Research Foundation
Holon 58484 (Israel)
E-Mail zfisman@post.tau.ac.il

Subject Index